trotman

getting into

School

Steven Piumatti

6th Edition

D1579184

Getting into Dental School

This 6th edition published in 2009 by Trotman Publishing, an imprint of Crimson Publishing Limited, Westminster House, Kew Road, Richmond, Surrey TW9 2ND

© Trotman Publishing 2009

Author Steven Piumatti

5th edn by James Burnett published in 2007
4th edn by James Burnett & Andrew Long published in 2005
3rd edn by James Burnett & Andrew Long published in 2003
2nd edn by Joe Ruston & James Burnett in 2000
1st edn by Joe Ruston in 1996

Editions 1–5 published by Trotman and Co Ltd

British Library Cataloguing in Publication Data
A catalogue record for this book is available from the British Library.

ISBN 978 1 84455 188 0

Typeset by IDSUK (Data Connection) Ltd.

Printed and bound in Great Britain by Bell & Bain Ltd, Glasgow

Table 4 (page 86) showing number of applicants to dental school reprinted with kind permission from UCAS.

Contents

About the author

Steven Piumatti is a Director of Studies and Careers Advisor at Mander Portman Woodward. He is in charge of the medical programme and runs work experience and interview preparation programmes for potential dentists and for dental students. He has also written the Trotman/MPW book *Getting into Medical School*.

Acknowledgements

This book would not have been possible without the help of many people. In particular, I would like to thank Dr Camisa, Dr Anne Aiken, Dr Neva Patel, Saba Saied, James Burnett, Maya Waterstone, Phillipa Brough, James Barton, Mr Kumal Datta, the dental students who helped to paint a picture of life at dental school, the admissions tutors from the dental schools who gave us the information on admissions, and the British Dental Association and British Dental Health Foundation for providing much of the factual material on careers in dentistry. However, I would like to emphasise that although the information in the book has been provided by experts, most of the views expressed are my own, and any mistakes are down to me.

Steven Piumatti
November 2008

For up-to-date information on dental schools, visit www.mpw.co.uk/ getintomed

About this book

This book is divided into nine chapters.

1| How to research your options
2| Studying dentistry
3| Your application and the personal statement
4| The interview stage and getting an offer
5| Results day
6| Non-standard applications
7| Careers in dentistry
8| Current issues/topics
9| Further information

Chapter 1 informs you on the need to get research done as early as possible and the possible steps that can be taken, while Chapter 2 describes the actual study of dentistry at undergraduate level and then beyond – like specialisations and possible post-degree options. Chapter 3 deals with the preparation that you will need to undertake in order to make your application as irresistible as possible. It includes advice on work experience, how to choose a dental school and the UCAS application procedure, and finishes with a checklist for you to tick off the important steps in making your application.

Chapter 4 provides advice on what to expect at the interview stage, and how to ensure that you come across as a potential dentist. Chapter 5 looks at the options you have on results day and describes the steps that you need to take if you are holding an offer, or if you do not have an offer, what then are your possible next steps. Chapter 6 is aimed primarily at overseas students who wish to apply and any other 'non-standard' applicants – mature students, graduates, students who have studied arts A levels and re-take students.

Chapter 7 looks at career options in dentistry and touches on the aspect of running a business, while Chapters 8 presents some key information on dental issues, such as fluoridation of water and the National Health Service (NHS) debate. Knowing about issues is a must, particularly if you are called in for an interview. Finally, in Chapter 9, further information is given via a series of tables.

Throughout the book you will find case studies and examples of material that will reflect to some extent the theme being discussed at that point. I hope that you find these real-life examples illuminating.

Like other books in this series, such as *Getting into Medical School*, this book is designed to be a route map for potential dentists, rather than a guide to dentistry as a profession. The British Dental Association, or your own dentist, should be the starting points for more detailed information on what being a dentist entails. For the latest news on dentistry and dental schools, visit www.mpw.co.uk/getintomed.

Entrance requirements have been given in terms of A level grades throughout the book; information for students who have studied Scottish Highers, the International Baccalaureate (IB) and other examinations is given on page 27.

Introduction

'Why would you want to spend all day looking into people's mouths? I can't think of anything worse!' This, typically, is the reaction when you tell someone that you want to become a dentist. The fact that you are reading this book probably means that you have realised that dentistry offers far more than this. What, then, are the attractions of a career and a life in dentistry?

The role of dentists in society

If you talk to dentists, they mention some or all of the following as being reasons why they chose dentistry:

- the opportunity to have day-to-day contact with a wide range of people
- an interest in human biology and dental issues
- freedom to choose your own patients
- an opportunity to run a business and be your own boss
- flexibility in choosing the length of the working day
- working as part of a team
- working with your hands, and being able to do so creatively
- being a positive and helpful part of the community
- helping and improving people's well-being, from the very young to the aged
- status and respect.

Dentistry is not just about teeth, but also about oral health in general. Dentists are increasingly becoming more than the narrow prescriptive role they once had. Today dentists have a wider role in society as oral professionals and also as health practitioners who look after the well-being of their patients. Through their work and advice they become role models in the community. The British Dental Health Foundation, which is associated with the International Health Foundation, has a very interesting website outlining the varied and wider role that dentists are expected to be familiar with these days. Visit www.dentalhealth.org.uk/faqs/browseleaflets.php to see the variety of angles and job demands that dentistry is required to fulfil these days. The roles vary from educational and advisory to surgical, and sometimes the role of a dietician. In the latter case dentists increasingly need to advise on what is healthy to eat and what is detrimental to your oral health, and in the long run to your overall health, confidence and well-being.

Have you considered, for example, some of the diverse situations that a dental practitioner has to be able to deal with, such as dental care for special needs? Patients with physical disabilities may have problems getting into the dental chair and people with learning disabilities may become distressed at the thought of going to the dentist and may need extra reassurance. Also people with severe medical problems may need extra precautions or care and a dentist must take account of all these things when providing dental care. In cases such as these, different arrangements have to be made by a practice/dentist, and often home visits may have to be organised. In the UK today, the Community Dental Service (CDS) is responsible for the treatment for people with learning difficulties or a medical disability. In such cases some dentists (or community dental officers) are willing to work in a more peripatetic fashion than in a full-time surgery environment, and the patient's dentist is responsible for referring them to the local clinic, with any hospital letters and X-rays, to give the community dental officer an idea of the patient's dental history.

Dentists need to know the patient's medical history and any medicines they are taking. This includes any inhalers and regularly prescribed medicines from a doctor. The dentist will also need to know the name of the family doctor, hospital consultant, and about any recent operations and allergies the patient may have. In addition, some patients may have other special needs, for example, an interpreter or translator, or the need for a guide dog. Therefore, dentists have to be prepared for working in a variety of different circumstances.

Another major aspect of the role in society that a dentist has is in terms of education. Along with dental nurses they are at the forefront of teaching the public how to brush their teeth and much more. There is a major push for preventive dentistry by the NHS and dentists today. It is about long-term care of the mouth, teeth, gums and cheeks, and extends, as previously mentioned, to areas such as diet. The teaching of awareness of oral health and hygiene is of paramount importance. Dentists educate patients on caring for teeth and gums by encouraging them to use fluorides, flossing and brushing. Teaching through direct consultations, and pamphlets often found in surgeries, is one way, with another way being the education of young people in schools and elderly people in nursing homes with regard to keeping dentures clean and viable. This is all carried out by dentists working within the CDS.

In this way, through preventive dentistry, the need for major dental treatment is kept to a minimum by maintaining a healthy mouth. As the two major causes of tooth loss are tooth decay and gum disease, the better we prevent or deal with these two problems, the more chance people have of keeping their teeth for life. The joint efforts of the dentist, the hygienist and the patient can help to prevent the need for treatment, and so avoid the traditional pattern of fillings and extractions, which is a saving not only to the individual in terms of time and money but also to the community in the long term.

Dentists are often the first to spot medical problems that might otherwise go unnoticed until the problem has worsened. An example of this is oral cancer. There are over 3,000 new cases of oral cancer each year, and about half of these patients die from the disease. This figure is comparable with more highly publicised cancers, such as skin cancer. Dentists are also the first people to recognise ulcers and cold sores that could lead to more serious problems. Like all disease, early recognition is more than half the battle.

A very interesting and recent development is the increasing use of dentists by the public for cosmetic improvement. This was an area of growth that was strongly commented on by the dentists with whom I spoke in researching this book. Not only is it increasing their scope but it is also a lucrative area in our image-conscious society. Cosmetic dental surgery involves treatments to straighten, lighten, reshape and repair teeth. This can also include veneers, crowns, bridges, tooth-coloured fillings, implants and tooth whitening and correction of bites. For example, as people get older, a face can sag, the chin can stick out and the smile droop if the 'bite' is not corrected – what dentists refer to as 'face collapse'. It can even cause headaches, neck pain and other pains in the body. Thus there is a need for rectification. Usually, obvious abnormal 'bites' or crooked teeth are fixed early in childhood but today even mild forms of the above are now seen as a problem and more young and mature adults than before are undergoing this type of cosmetic treatment.

Attributes of a dentist

Probably even more so than in medicine, candidates must be able to demonstrate not only academic ability and the right personal qualities, but also commitment. In researching this book, the dentists interviewed commented that commitment has to be paramount and evident. As dentistry is a much narrower field of science, a person must almost be 99% sure that he or she wants to become a dentist. This is because dentistry is such a specialised career that it is difficult once in it to be able to move effortlessly into something else without some degree of re-specialisation. So to go into dentistry because 'you like science' is frankly not enough. Dentistry, unlike medicine, offers fewer diverse pathways or opportunities later on, and thus a candidate must be all the more sure of what they are about to get into. Furthermore, dentistry requires a combination of many skills, and those applicants who cannot demonstrate these rarely get offers.

The main skills and personal qualities a dentist requires are:

- the ability to be reassuring, particularly to those who are scared or in pain
- an enjoyment of science and developments in the field of dentistry
- manual dexterity
- enjoyment of being around other people
- self-motivation
- a caring and sympathetic nature and immense patience
- an excellent memory
- versatility
- stamina – both mental and physical – remember a dentist may have to remain standing for hours
- the ability to work as part of a team
- the ability to multi-task – necessary for running a business
- ability to train and manage people and get the best out of them.

Some of the above qualities will not surprise you. It would be hard to be a successful dentist if you could not bear to be around other people, and unsympathetic dentists end up with few patients. Similarly, if you do not enjoy science, you would be unlikely to gain the necessary grades at A level, or to pass the dental school examinations. Also, and often overlooked, is the need for manual dexterity. If you think you have two left hands dentistry is probably not the course for you. The dentists I spoke to raised this point as one of great importance.

If you believe that you have the above qualities, the next step is to investigate what being a dentist is actually like, and find out what they do. In brief, a dentist's job includes tasks such as filling cavities, examining X-rays, applying protective sealant on teeth, extracting teeth, removing decay, and taking measurements and making models for dentures. They often treat gum disease by performing surgery on patients. As you can see, this is where versatility is needed – and stamina. Patience and empathy are also much-needed attributes, as every day a dentist will be working with patients and his or her staff.

Many people are unaware that dentists are usually self-employed, and the amount of money they earn is directly related to the number of patients they see. Without stamina, and the self-motivation to work hard without someone keeping an eye on you, you are unlikely, at least at the start of your career, to earn as much as you might hope. A survey by the British Dental Association (BDA) (2008) revealed that the average student debt on graduating was about £24,860 (not including mortgages) and a quarter of these students owed in excess of £30,000. Many of the students had multiple debts, including student loans, bank loans, overdrafts, credit cards and debt to parents. The most common types of debt were student and bank loans. Therefore, not surprisingly, once qualified, dentists need to earn enough not only to support themselves, but also to begin paying off their debts.

The downside

There are, of course, some negative aspects of dentistry. In its highly informative advice sheet on careers in dentistry, the BDA urges prospective dentists to consider a number of aspects including stress, lack of job and financial security (because of self-employment), lack of career progression, aggressive or frightened patients and, lastly, but by no means least, the boredom that can accompany repetitive routine tasks. If you are worried about any of these, you should talk to your own dentist to see how he or she feels about them. Some dentists will warn students against going into the profession without being aware that dentistry suits people who are prepared to work hard, and who enjoy being with other people.

Before looking at the applications and admissions processes in more detail, you may be interested to read what a recently commenced dental student had to say about his choice of career thus far. Bear in mind that this indeed could be you in one or two years' time.

Case study 1: A student

James Fenwick is currently studying dentistry at Liverpool University. A week's compulsory work experience while he was in Year 10 at school sparked an interest in the world of dentistry for James and he quickly came to appreciate the value of such an activity. This was not the natural route for James. His father had him marked down as a lawyer and to follow in his footsteps to the Square Mile. However, James was persuasive and a strong return in his GCSEs, and more importantly his A levels, meant that James joined Liverpool University this year as a dental undergraduate.

'While this was not necessarily the most obvious choice of careers for me, it was the one that I felt I could see myself doing. I could think of nothing worse than working in a city office grinding my fingers to the bone. Were it not for my work experience though, this choice might never have been brought to life. It is funny really how the decisions we make in life really do have a bearing on our future. As clichéd as that sounds, my work experience opened my eyes. The people were very friendly and eager to impress upon me the diversity that the profession can afford. I remember going from one extreme to another; watching with uncomfortable pleasure a root canal procedure to moulding a gum shield for a professional rugby club player. Every day afforded something new and while I appreciate that will not always be the situation in the profession, there is something to be said for treating patients on a case-by-case basis and taking a fresh approach each time.'

James' A level choices were influenced by his interest in the profession and he studied Biology, Chemistry and Physics and a further AS level in Theatre Studies. 'I was advised that my fourth AS subject was more for my interest rather than a necessity for my course so I choose Theatre Studies as I love to act. Admittedly Theatre Studies would appear to have no relevance to dentistry, however, in hindsight, what the course gave me was an incredible sense of confidence and belief in performing in front of people. I have never been a shy person but I was always guilty of not speaking out enough. While you are not expected to perform as a dentist – not unless you believe *Little Shop of Horrors* – you must have a calming influence as there are very few people who enjoy going to the dentist. I imagine it to be very much like being a doctor or a vet, because it makes your job a lot easier if your patient is relaxed.'

James' first semester in dentistry in Liverpool has been very hard and focused work so far and he has found it an enormous step up from his A level courses, something that he advises all aspiring dentists to be wary of. That, combined with a hectic social schedule, has meant that there is no rest for the wicked, but he is thoroughly enjoying this new challenge and he eagerly awaits the next four-and-a-half years. James would also like to point out that his forthcoming role as the sadistic dentist in *Little Shop of Horrors* is in no way intended as a faux pas and that he does maintain a healthy interest in other fields aside from dentistry, both academically and socially!

01 How to research your options

According to UCAS, in 2008 there were 2,737 applicants for entry into dentistry competing for 1,199 places, a ratio of 2.28 applicants per place. Of this, the ratio of women to men was about 55:44, and the ratio of places gained by women was slightly higher than men, with a success rate of 45% in comparison to 40%, respectively. In other words, women were on average slightly more successful than men in their applications. This might be due to an overall more mature approach, better preparation and focus and/or better AS grades overall.

Of these numbers approximately 350 were overseas applicants, of whom only 64 were accepted. Obviously, it is much more difficult to get a successful application through if you are an overseas applicant (see Chapter 6 for more information about this).

The 2008 numbers signal an increase in the number of applications from previous years so the forecast based on current trends is for application numbers to keep rising, thus increasing the competition for places and making AS grades and full preparation even more important in the coming years, as there will be more competition for the limited number of places available. Table 2 in Chapter 9 gives an indication of the 2008 and most recent 2009 application numbers, however, it does not give the number of places available as this information was not available at the time of writing. It is worth mentioning here that in the 2009 round of applications there was a 9.55% increase on the 2008 numbers to a total of 3,304. This figure includes both EU and non-EU applicants (see Table 4, Chapter 9).

Lastly, in 2008 there were approximately 90 students who narrowly missed their offers and therefore missed taking a place due to not gaining the necessary grades. Normally, under such circumstances in other courses, e.g. economics, these places would then be offered to prospective students immediately after results become available via the clearing system in mid August. However, a note of warning here is necessary, as all of the dental courses run by the universities do not take any students through clearing. This is because often the number of offers given in the first place is greater than the actual number of places. For example, a university may give 60 firm offers but yet only have 50 places. This is to ensure full capacity in the course and the number of offers takes into account students who do not get the required grades or who decide to go to another university.

Exploration of options

So what is it that you need to do to ensure that you have an excellent chance of getting selected for an interview and offered a place? (Not all universities will give interviews – most will offer places without interviews – see Table 1, Chapter 9).

The first step is to do your research as early as possible for the following reasons:

- to see if dentistry is really what you want to do
- to find out what university you will want to go to
- to find out what course each university offers and what might best suit you
- to research possible work experience/placements
- to find out the best way to set out a personal statement and practise for interviews.

Ideally you would have started your research in the AS year or even earlier. Most schools start the programme of UCAS and career prospects-related workshops half way through the AS year with the aim being that students should have a clear idea where they want to apply to after the summer holidays of the AS year, as they commence their A2 year.

There are several ports of call that students need to consider in their research. These can be divided into:

- media research – internet, books, periodicals and specialist magazines
- research via discussion with working professionals
- work experience.

With regard to the first bullet point, some suggestions are given below.

Internet

- The UCAS website (www.ucas.com) very useful for research into courses and universities.
- Newspaper sites – www.guardian.co.uk/education and *The Times* (www.timesonline.co.uk/education) which will take you to *The Times Good University Guide 2009*.
- www.mpw.co.uk/getintomed – this website will take to you links such as Department of Health and World Health Organization.
- Also very useful for researching this career is the BDA website (www.bda.org) and the British Dental Health Foundation website (www.dentalhealth.org.uk).
- www.dentistry.co.uk – this is an online periodical which is very useful for up-to-date information about the field of dentistry.

Books and periodicals

- *Degree Course Offers 2009*, 39th edition, by Brain Heap has a short section on dentistry and the universities offering dentistry courses.
- University prospectuses: calling universities and asking them to send you their prospectuses will help you get a feel for the university and the course.
- Subscribing to magazines such as *The Dentist* permits you to see at first hand the issues and developments in dentistry. This would be seen as extra-curricular reading and would show interest to prospective university panels.

Work experience

Discussing your interest in dentistry with dentists working in the field is an excellent idea. You might want to start with your own local dentist and ask him or her as much as you can think of regarding the career, including the positives and negatives of the job, the process of getting into university and any current and topical issues in dentistry. However, by far the best thing you can do to definitely find out if dentistry is for you is to organise either by yourself and/or via the school some work experience in a practice whereby you could shadow a dentist.

This is a vital part of your application – it is unlikely that you will be considered unless you have done so – but more importantly, it is a chance for you to see whether it is the right career for you. Whatever the attractions, if you cannot see yourself enjoying the job for the next 40 years, you should choose another career.

Most admissions tutors would agree that the absolute minimum amount of time that prospective dental students should spend work-shadowing dentists is two weeks – anything less than this will be unlikely to allow you to appreciate the realities of dentistry as a career. Ideally, you should aim to spend three or four weeks with one or more dentists, or to help out in a dental surgery on a regular basis over several months. The first thing to do is to arrange your work experience. If you are lucky, your school will have a scheme whereby it can arrange this for you, saving you the hard work of contacting dental practices. The disadvantage of this is that you will be unable to impress the selectors with your dynamism and determination because you will not be able to say 'I arranged my work experience myself.' If your school does not operate such a scheme, you have two options: to use any contacts that your family or friends have; or to approach local dentists. To do this, get the names and addresses of local dental practices from the telephone directory or the BDA (www.bda.org). You should write a formal letter, and include the name of a referee, someone who can vouch for your interest in dentistry as well as your reliability. Your careers teacher, housemaster/

housemistress or form teacher would be ideal. An example of a suitable letter is given below.

1 Melchester Road
Melchester
MC2 3EF
0123 456 7890

Mr P Mackie [Telephone the practice for the name of one of the dentists.]
Pain-free Dental Clinic
123 High Street
Melchester
MC1 1AB

1 October 2007

Dear Mr Mackie

I am in the first year of my A level studies, and I am interested in a career in dentistry. In order to find out more about dentistry, I would like to shadow a dentist, preferably for a week. I would be extremely grateful if you would be prepared to meet me, in order to discuss whether it would be possible for me to spend some time at the Pain-free Dental Clinic.

If you require a reference, please contact my careers teacher. His contact details are:

Mr N Townson, Head of Careers
Melchester High School
Melchester
MC1 2CD

I look forward to hearing from you.

Yours sincerely

L M Johnson

Lucy Johnson (Miss)

Shadowing dentists is useful for three reasons.

1| It will help you to decide whether you really want to be a dentist.
2| It will demonstrate your seriousness to admissions tutors.
3| You may, if you can demonstrate to the dentist that you are serious about dentistry, be able to ask him or her for a reference.

■ Things to look out for during work experience

The variety of treatments available to patients

Make sure that you know what you are observing. Ask the dentist or nurse for the technical names of the procedures that you see, and for information on the materials and equipment used. Ask about the advantages and disadvantages of different types of filling, implant or denture. Make sure that you are aware not only of how damaged teeth are repaired, but also about preventive dentistry, orthodontics and oral hygiene. You should also try to discuss the dentist's role in identifying other problems, such as mouth cancer.

Working as a dentist

Ask the dentist about his or her life. Find out about the hours, the way in which dentists are paid, the demands of the job, and the career options open to dentists. Find out what dentists like about the job, and what they dislike.

■ Tips for work experience

Dress as the dentists dress: be clean, tidy and reasonably formal.

Ask intelligent questions about the procedures that you witness, and keep a diary of the things that you see.

Offer to help the dentist or the receptionists with routine tasks.

Show an interest in all that is going on around you, bearing in mind that this might be your job in a few years' time. In the event that this work shadowing does not fulfil your expectations, you need to ask yourself why you would want to study this course.

Case study 2: Work experience

Mike studied at Leeds. He had wanted to be a doctor since he was 10, but when he was trying to get hospital work experience, his dentist suggested that Mike shadow him for a week. Mark quickly realised that he enjoyed the dentistry work experience much more than his medical placements, and he decided to change direction.

'I don't know what it was that made me decide on dentistry rather than medicine, but I came away from the dental practice each evening feeling excited, rather than depressed, as was happening when I shadowed doctors, who were all very negative about a career as a doctor. One of the things I particularly liked was how grateful the patients were, and how the dentist was able to build up a relationship

---

with them because he saw them on a regular basis. Doctors only see sick people!'

Mike was only made one offer, of ABB. In the end, he only achieved BBB but was accepted anyway, because he had performed well at the interview.

'I think it's fair to say that I made the most of my time at dental school. I played rugby and had a very good social life, as well as working very, very hard indeed. My aim is to own my own practice, somewhere in a big city. I like the idea of running a business, and I think that I would be good at it – I always enjoyed coming up with money-making schemes when I was at school.'

The BDA estimates that a dentist with no private patients earns, on average, about £100,000 a year. Dentists who offer private treatment generally earn more than this. Before you begin to think about how many Ferraris you could buy when you become a dentist, you should be aware that the expenses associated with running a practice can take more than 50% of this (on, for instance, wages, materials and the practice building). Even sole practitioners, who generally have greater control over the running of a practice, cannot expect to keep more than about 60% of their income. Another factor to consider is that, unlike other careers in which earnings rise year after year, dentists often reach a peak in their 30s, and their earnings can fall after this as they become older, slower and less inclined to work long hours.

02 Studying dentistry

Undergraduate

Dental courses are carefully planned to give students a wide range of academic and practical experience that will lead to final qualification as a dentist. At the end of the five-year course students will, if they have met the high academic standards demanded, be awarded a Bachelor of Dental Surgery (referred to as either BDS or a BChD, depending on which dental school you are at).

The structure of all dental courses is similar, with most institutions offering two years of pre-clinical studies (often undertaken with medical students at the same university) followed by three years of clinical studies. The pre-clinical studies are often taught outside the dentistry school, with regular visits to the school forming part of the learning programme. However, every school differs in the way in which it delivers the material so it is very important to get hold of, and thoroughly read, the latest prospectuses. For example, here are two descriptions of a degree in dentistry. The first one – from Leeds – seems to have a more holistic approach.

Programme structure - Leeds (2008)

'A broad range of learning and teaching methods are used including lectures, seminars, tutorials, e-learning, reflective learning and group projects.

The programme takes an integrated approach, i.e. the courses do not focus on a specific subject but cover areas such as Health and Health Promotion, Oral Disease, Defence and Repair, Anxiety and Pain Management and Wellbeing and Illness, Social Context of Disease. Emphasis is placed upon contextualised and relevant learning and students will gain clinical experience from Year 1. There are several themes running throughout the programme including Communications Skills, Personal and Professional Development, Working as a Member of a Team and Clinical Practice and Outreach. Various optional courses such as Psychology in Dentistry, Modern Languages, Advanced Restorative Dentistry and Law, Ethics and Morality will be available in Years 4 and 5.'

Source: www.ucas.com

Compare the Leeds brief with the one from the University of Birmingham.

Programme structure - Birmingham (2008)

'Your degree consists of five terms of pre-clinical studies followed by three years and one term of clinical work. The pre-clinical programme in your first and second years is modular in form and based on the interdisciplinary study of the different systems of the body, with subjects including anatomy, physiology, biochemistry, oral biology and pharmacology. The emphasis is on small group teaching and self-learning.

There are modules on Biological Sciences and on the Principles of Learning. You also take modules on Clinical Dentistry and Behavioural Science in preparation for your first contact with patients. This takes place early in this year.

The clinical programme covers specialist subjects such as paediatric dentistry, restorative dentistry, dental prosthetics, and oral medicine and surgery. You extend your practical experience with the clinical practice programme. Here, you take responsibility for your own patients' treatment by running what amounts to your own mini-practice within the Dental Hospital. In this way you learn to apply specialist teaching within the framework of whole-patient care and teamwork.

Alongside your clinical work you continue with programmes in oral biology and pathology. As part of your study of medicine and surgery you spend some of your time in residence at a general hospital. You learn about the social and psychological side of patient care while developing your interpersonal and communication skills. You also gain an appreciation of the factors involved in controlling dental disease, together with epidemiology and statistical techniques, and key ethical and medico-legal issues that surround the practice of dentistry.

As you near the end of your clinical course you have time to pursue your own elective programme of study a topic of personal interest, which you research on your own.

Your final year of study consists of a common core of academic work and clinical dental practice. You may also select a special study module for in-depth work.'

Source: www.ucas.com

Universities teach in a range of ways, from traditional large lectures to small tuition groups of approximately eight. A number of schools, such as Liverpool and Manchester, have successfully used a problem-based learning (PBL) approach which, they feel, encourages the students to develop an independent and inquisitive approach to learning, using libraries and discussing issues with colleagues to solve problems (as the name suggests). Some schools stress the importance of contact with the patient very early in the course while others prefer students to finish the pre-clinical course before this happens. All the schools are very interested in embracing the latest technologies using both com-puter modelling and the simulation of procedures and techniques using, for instance, a 'phantom head'.

The reason why a dental course lasts five years is that the teaching cov-ers a wide variety of elements. The pre-clinical students will typically study some, or all, of the following courses: anatomy; biomedical sci-ences; physiology; biochemistry; oral biology; pharmacology; first aid; and an introduction to the clinical skills that will be taught later in the course. In addition, students will cover the effects of anaesthetics and other components common to medicine and dentistry. Furthermore, aspects of psychology will also be considered because dentists work in close proximity with people and use skills and techniques to relax patients.

Specialisation and hands-on training are provided in the last year. Spe-cialisation includes orthodontics, periodontics, oral pathology, oral surgery, operative dentistry and prosthodontics. The postgraduate course in dentistry (Master of Dental Science) has a two-year duration and offers several specialties.

Students who perform well in the examinations at the end of the pre-clinical course (Year 2) often take up the opportunity to complete an intercalated BSc. This is normally a one-year project, during which stu-dents have the opportunity to investigate a chosen topic in much more depth, producing a written thesis before rejoining the course.

When clinical studies start (Years 3, 4 and 5), students often take respon-sibility for their own patients in the in-house 'mini-practices' or as part of a team comprising students of varied experience (in some schools this includes training with chair-side assistants, dental technicians and hygien-ists). Students are also encouraged to participate in practitioner attach-ment schemes in which they spend time with general dental practitioners (GDPs), specialist dental units and the CDS. Time can also be spent at local hospitals to gain experience of accident and emergency, general, and ear, nose and throat surgery. To teach the patient care necessary to effectively treat a range of people, many schools are now offering courses in behavioural sciences and the management of pain and anxi-ety, as well as in the treatment of children, and elderly and disabled people. The clinical students will typically study some of the following courses: behavioural science; computing and statistics; dental materials; dental public health; dental prosthetics; haematology; operative tech-nique and clinical skills; children's dentistry; restorative dentistry; oral medicine and surgery; oral pathology; oral biochemistry and biology; orthodontics; medico-legal and ethical aspects of dental practice; forensic dentistry; sedation; radiology and other aspects of the management of pain and anxiety in dentistry.

Towards the end of the course there is often the opportunity to take an elective study period, when students are expected to undertake a short project but are free to travel to any hospital or clinic in the world that is approved by their university. For example, Bristol Dental School has links with, among others, Bordeaux, Paris and Valencia, and less formal links with other parts of the world. A number of dental schools have excellent working links with European universities. This means that under the Socrates–Erasmus scheme a limited number of students study at another participating European university and are credited with the academic work they undertake there.

At the end of Year 5 there is the final BDS/BChD professional examination. The dental schools include all clinical aspects of dentistry in their courses, which means that graduates are competent to carry out most treatments and exercise independent clinical judgement.

Postgraduate

According to the British Council there is a wide variety of opportunities for further postgraduate education and training in dentistry. However, before any form of clinical training can commence (i.e. training involving hands-on contact with patients), dental graduates must register with the General Dental Council.

Dental schools/hospitals run a wide range of postgraduate programmes which include further clinical and non-clinical training and research degree programmes. Advice and guidance are available from the National Advice Centre for Postgraduate Dental Education (NACPDE). Information on postgraduate courses can be found on the NACPDE website (www.rcseng.ac.uk/fds/nacpde). As before, what you will need to do is check the prospectuses of individual universities for the most up-to-date information.

Here is an example of postgraduate courses, taken from the Manchester University website.

- Control of Pain and Anxiety (including Conscious Sedation) Hypnosis
- Dental Implantology
- Endodontics
- Fixed and Removable Prosthodontics
- Oral and Maxillofacial Surgery
- Orthodontics
- Masters in Public Health and Primary Care

In addition, universities offer research opportunities. Manchester Dental School, for example, offers a doctorate in a variety of streams, such as in Clinical Dental Science, a two-year course leading to a Clinical PhD. Moreover, continuous professional development (CPD) is also offered in many universities. These are courses for qualified dentists who want to develop their knowledge of the latest methods, equipment and techniques. Manchester University, a case in point, 'offers hands-on training and three hours of verifiable CPD in a world-class environment.' (Source: www.dentistry.manchester.ac.uk/postgraduate/cpd/)

Postgraduate courses, particularly master's and courses leading to doctorates, are not cheap, particularly for overseas students/dentists.

Specialisms

The following sections briefly look at the major specialisations in dentistry.

Restorative dentistry

Restorative dentistry is the study, diagnosis and effective management of diseases of the teeth and their supporting structures. Restorative dentistry falls under three categories: prosthodontics, periodontology and endodontology.

- **Endodontics** is the branch of dentistry that concerns itself with dealing with health and injuries and diseases of the pulp and periradicular region (the tooth root and its surrounding tissue), such as root canal injuries, which can harm the nervous system as well.
- **Periodontics** is the branch of dentistry dealing with the supporting structures of teeth and includes the treatment of patients with severe gum disease.
- **Prosthodontics** deals mainly with the replacement of hard and soft tissues using crowns, bridges, dentures and implants. It focuses on treatment planning, rehabilitation and maintenance of the oral function, comfort and appearance.

Paediatric dentistry

Paediatric dentistry is the practice, teaching, and research into oral health care for children from birth to adolescence. Children are unique in their stages of development, oral disease and oral health needs, and this is why paediatric dentistry covers all aspects of oral health care for children. It aims to improve oral health in children and encourage the highest standards of clinical care. According to the BDA, research has shown that children who visit paediatric dentists are far less likely to require a repeat general anaesthetic for further dental treatment.

Oral surgery

Oral surgery is surgery to correct a wide spectrum of diseases, injuries and defects in the head, neck, face, jaws and the hard and soft tissues of the oral and maxillofacial region. It is a recognised international surgical specialty. Oral surgery is a slightly more intrusive form of surgery than typical root canal or cavity fillings. It usually requires the use of anaesthetic and therefore patients take longer to recover. Examples of oral surgery include having your wisdom teeth removed and getting dental implants.

Dental public health

Dental public health is a non-clinical specialty which includes assessment of dental health needs and ensuring that dental services meet those needs. It is mainly concerned with improving the dental health of a population rather than that of individuals and it involves working in primary care trusts, government offices and strategic health authorities. There are a few academic posts in universities and in the Department of Health.

Orthodontics

Orthodontics is a specialty of dentistry that is centred on the study and treatment of malocclusions (improper bites), which may result in tooth irregularity, out-of-proportion jaw relationships, or both. Orthodontic correction has a very positive effect on facial appearance.

Oral medicine

This is concerned with the diagnosis and non-surgical management of medical pathology affecting the oral area, jaw and face. Many oral medicine specialists have dual qualifications, with both medical and dental degrees. The main aspects of oral medicine are clinical care, research and undergraduate and postgraduate teaching.

Oral microbiology

This is the study of bacteria in our mouths. The mouth has a diverse and complex microbial community. Bacteria accumulate on both the hard and soft oral tissues. There is a highly developed defence system that monitors the bacteria colonisation and prevents bacteria invasion of local tissues.

Oral pathology

Oral pathology is the branch of dentistry concerned with the diseases of oral structures, including soft tissues, teeth, jaws and salivary glands. Oral pathology is a science that investigates the causes, processes and effects of these diseases. The practice of oral pathology includes research and diagnosis of diseases using clinical, radiographic and biochemical means.

Forensic odontology

This is a relatively new and very exciting branch of dentistry, not least because of the plethora of *CSI* and *Waking the Dead* type programmes on television. This branch of dentistry deals with the proper handling and examination of dental evidence, followed by the evaluation of said evidence. It involves the identification either through ante- or post-mortem means of the causes of death or establishing vicinity and proof in a crime, for example, in the comparison of bite-marks on victims of assault and rape.

Dental and maxillofacial radiology

Dental and maxillofacial radiology involves a combination of radiology and dentistry. It is mainly concerned with using and understanding diagnostic imaging modalities used in dentistry.

Prosthetics

Prosthetics is the science that is concerned with the diagnosis, prevention and treatment of the diseases of the teeth, gums, and related structures of the mouth, including the repair of replacement or defective teeth. The main areas that are covered by prosthetic dentistry are crowns (which provide full coverage restoration of the tooth), bridges (which replace a missing tooth or teeth), dentures (which replace missing teeth or full arch) and implants (which replace one or more missing teeth).

Cosmetic dentistry

The focal point of this type of dentistry involves improvements in appearance either following trauma such as an accident or for perceived or real improvements in appearance for a beautiful and healthy smile. This involves teeth whitening, tooth decorations (jewellery), cosmetic white fillings and cosmetic ceramic rims.

■ Fees and funding

To find out the fees and funding for dentistry courses, prospective students should explore each of the universities' websites and/or talk to their financial departments. This is because fees and funding procedures vary from university to university.

Whether undertaking undergraduate or postgraduate studies, the costs can be considerable. As stated earlier and by the BDA, student debt was anywhere between £18,000 and £30,000. Bear in mind that the difference depends on many factors. Factors affecting the overall debt can range from geographical – does the student live in a city or not? Or the amount of help that parents can give. Is there a scholarship? And/or has the student has found some work? Whatever the circumstances, a student must give serious consideration to the cost and be prepared to fully commit. It also has to involve careful financial planning for the four or five years that a course may last. On top of the tuition fees students will also have to consider living costs. Needless to say in big cities like London, living costs will be much higher than in other parts of the country. One estimate is that London will cost about £9,000pa to cover food, accommodation, travel and books.

Home students, that is UK nationals and EU students, pay lower tuition fees than non-EU/UK students. For international students from outside these two regions, the costs can be prohibitive. At King's College, London, for example, the overseas tuition fees in 2008/09 will be £11,550 per year for the classroom-based programmes (this is the pre-clinical two-year course); for the subsequent three years, the clinically based programme is £26,900 per year. This is part of the reason why there are so few oversees students studying dentistry in the UK.

To use another example, this time at Birmingham University, the fees for overseas students in the academic year 2008/09 are as follows (source: www.international.bham.ac.uk/fees_faq.htm#1):

- non-lab fee (i.e. pre-clinical): £9,450
- laboratory fee (for programmes involving significant laboratory or workshop-based activities): £12,250
- clinical fee (for the clinical years of programmes in the Schools of Medicine and Dentistry): £22,350.

For UK students the fees are much lower. They also have the added advantage that they are eligible for a tuition fees loan or a student loan.

Student grants

Home students' grants in 2009 can help with the paying of tuition fees, but this depends on an assessments made by the local authority on how much a student's parents earn. A student will only get a full grant if the assessment comes to £25,000 or less.

Student loans

The most common way that students can fund themselves is by taking out a student loan. Students can take out two types of loan: loan for fees and loan for living costs. Students only start repaying these loans once they have finished studying and are earning over £15,000 per year.

NHS bursaries

In 2009, NHS bursaries are expected to be available for full- and part-time students. To be eligible for such a bursary, a student must qualify as a 'home student' and be on a course which is accepted as an NHS-funded place. These bursaries will be available for dentistry as it is recognised as a NHS-funded course. For more information, see the NHS students' grants unit website (www.nhsstudentgrants.co.uk). It is not surprising that many students take up paid work during the vacations or at weekends. It is also worth finding out from universities if scholarships are available.

03 Your application and the personal statement

In order to gain a place at dental school, you have to submit a UCAS application. Before you do this, however, you need to be sure that you have investigated the field of dentistry as thoroughly as you can. Most people have (or think that they have) a good idea about medicine as a career because it gets wide publicity. Almost every night, there is a medical programme on television – *Casualty*, *Holby City*, *ER*, *Grey's Anatomy* and *Green Wing*, to name but a few – but there is considerably less exposure to dentistry. How many films can you name that feature dentists? Most people can only get as far as Laurence Olivier in *Marathon Man* – not an ideal role model! On TV, Kyle MacLachlan in *Desperate Housewives* and Robert Lindsay in *My Family* also portray very flawed characters.

It is also fair to say that dentistry is a narrower profession than medicine, and it is vital that you are aware of what being a dentist entails on a day-to-day basis before committing yourself. This is not to say that all dentists do the same thing. As we shall see later, dentistry offers a variety of career paths, but there are fewer options available to dentists than to doctors.

Choice of school

Once you have completed your work experience, and are sure that you want to be a dentist, you need to research your choice of dental school. There are various factors that you should take into account:

- the type of course
- the academic requirements
- location
- whether the dental school is part of a large university, or a stand-alone medical and dental school.

The next step is to get hold of the prospectuses. If your school does not have spare copies, call the dental schools and they will send you copies free of charge. Most dental schools have very informative websites that carry extra information on admissions policies. At the end of the book, there is a list of the major dental organisations in the UK from which you can procure further information and a list of the 14 dental schools, complete with the names and contact details of the admissions tutors and/or admissions secretary in each of the universities. It would be worthwhile to make contact with as many of these as possible or at least with the ones that you have applied to.

Once you have narrowed down the number of dental schools to, say, six or seven, you should try to visit them in order to get a better idea of what studying there will be like. Your school careers department will have details of open days (or you could call the dental schools directly), and some schools can arrange for you to be shown around at other times of the year as well. Do not simply select a dental school because someone has told you that it has a good reputation or that it is easier to get into. You will be spending the next five years of your life at one of them, and if you do not like the place, you are unlikely to last the course.

Apart from talking to current or ex-dental students or careers advisers, there are a number of other sources of information (already mentioned in previous chapters) that will help you in making your choice. The *Guardian* and *The Times* publish their own league tables of dental schools, ranked by a total score that combines a number of assessment categories, including teaching scores, student–staff ratios and job prospects. The 2008 *Guardian* table placed Dundee first, followed by Leeds, Queen Mary, Sheffield and Cardiff, while *The Times* placed Sheffield first, followed by Glasgow, Queen Mary, King's, Leeds and Dundee. Of course, there is no such thing as a bad dental school in the UK, and league tables only tell you a small part of the whole story. They are based on a range of variables and this is why there is a discrepancy between the tables of the two newspapers.

Remember that league tables are no substitute for visiting the dental schools, looking at the course content in detail, and reading the prospectuses.

■ Academic requirements

In addition to the grades required at A level, all of the dental schools specify the minimum grades that they require at GCSE. This varies from dental school to dental school, but it is unlikely that you will be considered unless you have at least five A or A* grades, with at least B grades in Science, English and Mathematics. If your grades fall below these requirements, your referee will need to comment on them to explain why you underperformed (due to illness, family disruption, etc.) and/or why they expect your A level performance to be better than your GCSE grades indicate.

If you are worried about achieving the right grades, you should think carefully about choosing at least two dental schools that accept re-take candidates. Tables 1 and 2 in Chapter 9 give further information on this and show which dental schools consider students who have not achieved the minimum grades at the first attempt. The reason for including two (or more) of these dental schools is that many places will give preference to students who applied there first time round. Some even specify it as a requirement for re-takers.

In addition to specifying A level grades, some dental schools will ask for a minimum grade in the free-standing AS level. At the moment this is usually a B grade. Just as important is the fact that AS levels contribute 50% to the total A level score, and poor AS level grades will make it difficult, if not impossible, to achieve A grades at A level. AS level grades also give admissions tutors more to go on than GCSE grades and A level predictions alone, since the AS grades will be published in the August preceding your UCAS application and will feature on it. For the student, this means that the first year of A levels is as important as the second.

The typical entry grade requirements of the dental schools are shown in Tables 1 and 2 in Chapter 9. You should also check the schools' prospectuses for details of GCSE requirements and AS level requirements. Some dental schools specify that they require one of the AS subjects to be an arts or humanities subject, rather than all of them being sciences or mathematics.

Other qualifications

If you are not studying A levels, you should check with each dental school about their requirements. Listed below is a rough indication of what they might ask for.

- **Scottish Highers**: AAAAA–AABBB at Advanced Higher/Higher level. Higher level Chemistry and Biology are required, with at least one at Advanced Higher level.
- **International Baccalaureate**: 6, 6, 5 and 35–36 points overall. Chemistry plus one other science or mathematical subject to be taken at Higher level with passes in English and Mathematics at Standard level.
- **European Baccalaureate**: 80% overall, with 80% in each science option; chemistry and another science as full options.

You will need to check each university for the above entry requirements as there is some variation in their demands.

Non-dental choices

There are six spaces on the UCAS application, but only four of these can be used to select dentistry courses. The remaining spaces either can be left blank or can be filled with other choices. Whatever you do, do not put down medicine or veterinary science as your fifth and sixth choices, because not only will the medical school or veterinary school reject you, but it will be obvious to the selectors that you are not committed to dentistry. You are allowed to choose courses such as dental hygiene or dental therapy, but this is also not a good idea since students who take alternative dental courses tend to get frustrated and drop out. If you decide that you would be happy to accept an alternative to dentistry if you are unsuccessful, by all means choose another course, as long as you feel able to justify the choice at interview. However, my advice is to leave it blank because:

- it demonstrates to the selectors that you are committed to becoming a dentist
- you do not run the risk of feeling obliged to accept a place on a course that you do not wish to take.

■ UKCAT

Some dental schools now require applicants to sit the UKCAT (United Kingdom Clinical Aptitude Test) before they apply. The dental schools currently using the test are Cardiff, Dundee, Glasgow, King's, Manchester, Newcastle, Queen Mary, Queen's University Belfast and Sheffield. Registration for the 2009 test (for applicants applying for 2010 entry) starts in the first week of June 2009 and ends on 31 August 2009. You must take the test before the deadline of 10 October 2009. You need to register online at www.ukcat.ac.uk and sit the test at an external test centre. The cost for those who took the test in 2008 was £60 for candidates taking the test in the EU before 31 August 2008 and £95 for other candidates. Between 1 September and 10 October 2008 the cost was £75 for candidates taking the UKCAT in the EU. The costs are not envisaged to change in 2009. The 2008 test lasted two hours and consisted of five sections:

- verbal reasoning
- quantitative reasoning
- abstract reasoning
- decision analysis
- non-cognitive component.

Although the UKCAT website tries to discourage students from doing any preparation for the test other than taking the practice test available on the website, students who sat it in 2006 found that the more practice they had on timed IQ-type tests, the better prepared they felt. The reference section of most bookshops has a number of books that contain practice questions of a similar type to the UKCAT. Some useful titles are listed on the website that accompanies this book (www.mpw.co.uk/getintomed).

Personal statement

In order to increase access to dental treatment in the UK, the government announced in 2006 a new dental school at the Peninsula Medical School (which will offer four-year courses for science graduates and health care professionals) with 100 new dental training places shared between Peninsula, Liverpool University, Leeds University and Exeter University. King's and Manchester University also run a four-year graduate entry programme aimed at biomedical or health-related graduates.

So while this is good news, the problem is that, as previously stated, the number of candidates applying has also gone up. So what does the recent rise in applicants for dentistry mean? Almost certainly, that the grade requirements for entry into dental school will also continue to rise, and in order to differentiate between applicants, universities will set very high entry requirements. In the late 1990s, when application numbers were lower, candidates often received BBC offers, whereas now the standard offer is likely to be AAB or even AAA, and if you are a re-take candidate then you are most likely to be asked for AAA.

Consequently, when your UCAS application is received by the dental school, it will not be on its own but in a batch, possibly of many. The selectors will have to consider it, along with the rest, in between the demands of other aspects of their jobs. If your application is badly worded, uninteresting or lacking the things that the selector feels are important, it will be put on the 'reject without interview' pile. A typical dental school might receive 800 applications, which have to be reduced to 300 to be called for interview. You can only be called for interview on the basis of your UCAS application and so the more thought that you give to your UCAS application the better it will be and the higher chance that you will either be offered a conditional place or asked to come in for an interview. Remember that the selectors will not know about the things that you have forgotten to say and they can only get an impression of you from what is in the application. I have come across too many good students who never got an interview, simply because they did not think properly about their UCAS application: they relied on their hope that the selectors would somehow see through the words and get an instinctive feeling about them.

Note: it is not necessary that all candidates be interviewed. The number of those interviewed depends on the university. Tables 1 and 2 in Chapter 9 provide an outline of the percentage and numbers in real terms that dental schools interview. For example, the interview policy at Bristol is around 40% of those who apply, which in 2008 translated to about 220 interviews.

Almost all applicants now submit their applications via 'Apply' on www. ucas.com; follow the instructions and use the drop-down menus and help features to avoid errors. This can be completed on any computer linked to the internet and the application can be forwarded to your referee very easily.

The following sections will tell you more about what the selectors are looking for in a personal statement, and how you can avoid common mistakes. However, before looking at how the selectors go about deciding who to call to interview, there are several important things that you need to think about.

Therefore, your personal statement is of paramount importance as this is your chance to show the university selectors three very important themes. These are:

1| why you want to be a dentist?
2| what have you done to investigate the profession?
3| and lastly . . . are you the right sort of person for their dental school? In other words what are your personal qualities that make you an outstanding candidate?

The personal statement is your opportunity to demonstrate to the selectors that you have not only researched dentistry thoroughly, but also have the right personal qualities to succeed as a dentist. Do not be tempted to write the statement in the sort of formal English that you find in, for example, job applications. Read through a draft of your statement, and ask yourself the question 'Does it sound like me?' If not, rewrite it. Avoid phrases such as 'I was fortunate enough to be able to shadow a dentist . . .' when you really just mean 'I shadowed a dentist . . .' or 'I arranged to shadow a dentist . . .'.

Why dentistry?

A high proportion of UCAS applications contain a phrase such as 'From an early age I have wanted to be a dentist because it is the only career that combines my love of science with the chance to work with people.' Admissions tutors not only get bored with reading this, but it is also clearly untrue: if you think about it, there are many careers that combine science and people, including teaching, pharmacy, physiotherapy and nursing. However, the basic ideas behind this sentence may well apply to you. If so, you need to personalise it. You could mention an incident that first got you interested in dentistry – a visit to your own dentist, a conversation with a family friend, or a lecture at school, for instance. You could write about your interest in human biology or a biology project that you undertook when you were younger to illustrate your interest in science, and you could give examples of how you like to work with others. The important thing is to back up your initial interest in dentistry with your efforts to investigate the career.

What have you done to investigate dentistry?

This is where you describe your work experience. It is important to demonstrate that you gained something from the work experience, and that it has given you an insight into the profession. You should give an indication of the length of time that you spent at each dental practice, what treatments you observed, and your impressions of dentistry. You could comment on what aspects of dentistry attract you, what you found interesting or on something that surprised you.

Here is an example of a description of a student's work experience that would *not* impress the selectors:

> '*I spent three days at my local dental practice. I saw some patients having fillings, and a man whose false teeth didn't fit. It was very interesting.*'

The example below would be much more convincing because it is clear that the student is interested in what was happening.

> '*During my two weeks at the Pain-free Dental Clinic, I shadowed two dentists and a hygienist. I watched a range of treatments including fillings, a root canal, extractions and orthodontic treatment. I found particularly interesting the fact that, although both dentists had very different personalities, they both related well to the patients, who seemed to find them very reassuring. A number of things surprised me, in particular, how demanding a dentist's day is.*'

With luck, the selectors may pick on this at interview, and ask questions about the methods that the dentists used to relax their patients, or the demands of dentistry.

Personal qualities

As a dentist, you will be working with others throughout your career. To qualify as a dentist, you will study alongside possibly 50 others in your year, for five years. The person reading your UCAS application has to decide two things: whether you have the right personal qualities to become a successful dentist, and whether you will cope with and contribute to dental school life. To be a successful dentist, you need to be able to:

- relate to other people
- survive and enjoy dental school
- get on with a wide range of people.

Unlike school life, where many of the activities are organised and arranged by the teachers, almost all of the social activities at university are instigated and organised by students. For this reason, the selectors are looking for people who have the enthusiasm and ability to motivate others and to be prepared to give up their own time to arrange sporting, dramatic, musical or social activities.

How, then, does the person reading your personal statement know whether you have the qualities that they are looking for? They will expect to read about some of the following:

- participation in team events
- involvement in school plays or concerts
- positions of responsibility
- work in the local community
- part-time or holiday jobs
- ability to get on with people
- manual dexterity.

Weak and strong personal statements – exemplars

Below is an example of a personal statement that would be considered weak and would be unlikely to lead to an offer being made.

Personal statement: Example 1 (word count: 260)

I have chosen to study dentistry at university because I want to work with people and run a dentistry practice at some point in the future. I think that I am a fairly good manager of people and have good skills, and like science very much. I first became interested in dentistry because my uncle runs a practice and so I was able to see what is needed in the running of such a business. I spent a lot of time in the practice as a young child and have also worked for him.

Last summer, I spent two weeks shadowing a dentist in the local CDS, and I gained an insight into the skills required to be a successful dentist. In particular, I observed the need for good communication skills with patients. I enjoy reading *The Dentist* and sometimes the *BMJ*.

I am studying Chemistry, Biology and Economics at A level. Economics is useful because it helps me to understand supply and demand and will give me insights hopefully in how to run a business. Biology and Chemistry have both given me analytical skills and the ability to solve problems.

At school, I am captain of the football team. This requires the ability to show leadership qualities. It also allows me to get rid of stress. I play the piano and have been in the school band. This involves teamwork and manual dexterity. I like reading and travelling, and even cooking. On Saturdays, I work for GAP clothes store and so I have gained excellent communication and teamwork skills.

Personal statement: Example 1 raises a number of points.

1| It is too short, fewer than 300 words. You have enough space for 610–620 words and you should aim to use the full amount of space available.

2| Although the candidate has addressed all of the relevant issues and has three clear sections, there is a lack of detail. It is too general and tells us very little about the candidate.

3| It is generic and very not very personal. This is a chance for you to show how you are different from the hundreds of other candidates who apply and there should be an attempt to have some anecdotal evidence about who you are.

The weaknesses identified above can be rectified with a lot more thought and effort being given to the personal statement.

Section 1

I have chosen to study dentistry at university because I want to work with people and run a dentistry practice at some point in the future. I think that I am a fairly good manager of people and have good skills and like science very much. [*Give an example of why.*] I first became interested in dentistry because my uncle runs a practice and so I was able to see what is needed in the running of such a practice. I spent a lot of time in the practice as a young child and have also worked for him. [*Again, give an example of what in particular drove you to dentistry.*]

Section 2

Last summer, I spent two weeks shadowing a dentist in the local CDS, [*Give details about the practice – What type is it? Where? And what is CDS – Don't assume that readers will know*] and I gained an insight into the skills [*such as . . .*] required to be a successful dentist. In particular, I observed the need for good communication skills with patients. [*Again give an example of why these are important, such as describing a situation that you observed.*] I enjoy reading *The Dentist* and sometimes the *BMJ*. [*This should be the strongest and longest section. I want to know much more about what you gained from the work experience and why it has convinced you that your choice is the right one.*]

Section 3

I am studying Chemistry, Biology and Economics at A level. Economics is useful because it helps me to understand supply and demand and will give me insights hopefully in how to run a business. Biology and Chemistry have both given me analytical skills and the ability to solve problems.

At school, I am captain of the football team. This requires the ability to show leadership qualities. It also allows me to get rid of stress. I play the piano and have been in the school band. This involves teamwork and manual dexterity. I like reading and travelling, and even cooking. On Saturdays, I work for GAP clothes store and so I have gained excellent communication and teamwork skills. [*This is OK but could do with links between what you have studied at a level, and what you have discovered about dentistry in the real world through reading and work experience.*]

Here are two examples of much better personal statements. The first one has been broken down into sections with headings and the second one shows variations on a theme. Both demonstrate clarity and focus and what comes through is the enthusiasm that the candidates have for dentistry. These will give the applicant an excellent chance of being called in for an interview and being given an offer.

Example 2 has been broken down into the three or so sections usually used in a strong personal statement. Each of these three sections delivers and focuses on different themes, and is an integral component of the statement, which when combined together make an overall notable personal statement.

Personal statement: Example 2 (word count: 381)

Why I chose dentistry

My interest in dentistry started when my local dentist came to my school to give a careers talk. Until that point, my view of dentistry was based on my own nervousness when I visited the dentist. However, the talk showed me that there was more to dentistry than simply filling cavities. I began to realise that dentistry involved an understanding of science, an ability to keep up to date with new technologies, and a chance to run a business, as well as allowing me to use my communication skills.

Work experience

I spent two weeks shadowing my local dentist. During this time, the dental nurse was away for a day, so I was able to help the dentist with simple tasks such as sterilising instruments. I was also able to help the receptionist with filing and talking to patients in the waiting room. This showed me the need for sensitivity and confidentiality. I was also able to discuss what dentistry as a career involves. I enjoyed my time at the Pain-free Dental Clinic, and so I arranged to get a Saturday job at another local dental practice, helping the nurse. I have been doing this for nine months. The dentist let me practise using the drill on some extracted teeth, and I realised that it was much more difficult than it looked. I was very interested in finding out about what the dentist thought about the new NHS reforms and whether they were likely to improve working conditions for dentists and the availability of treatment for patients.

Activities and responsibilities

I am head of my form at school, which involves working with the teachers to ensure that everything runs smoothly. I play football for the 1st XI and cricket for the 2nd XI. I play the clarinet in the school orchestra, and for relaxation I am learning to play the guitar. As well as my Saturday job, I go to my local old people's home once a week to talk to the residents. As part of the school charity committee, I have helped to organise a sponsored fast, which raised £986 for Shelter. I enjoy going out with my friends at the weekend, and am planning to travel around Europe with three of them during the summer.

Personal statement: Example 3 (word count: 610)

Dentistry has been my key interest since I observed an extraction in a general practice while on work experience. I was mesmerised by the skill and speed displayed and how easy and painless modern dental technology had made this extraction process. I was particularly intrigued by the speed with which an upper wisdom tooth could be extracted. During my work experience at an orthodontic clinic I increased my understanding about why extractions are required somewhat less frequently now than in the past because of advances in orthodontic techniques. Through all my additional work experience over 2008 I became certain that this was what I wanted to do.

Dentistry combines my interest in science and my enjoyment of art, working with my hands, and, above all, working with people. So I am applying now before going on my gap year. I have planned work experience in a dental practice in New Zealand, and after reading *Oral Health in Uganda: The Need for a Change in Focus* by L B Muhirwe (*International Dental Journal* 2006), I am keen to see how dentistry is practised in developing countries, particularly in South East Asia.

Chemistry at A level has helped me develop a methodical approach to situations and taught me the importance of attention to detail. While working at the orthodontic clinic, I practised being meticulous when I learnt about the Index of Orthodontic Treatment Needed and to sort people into classes depending on their dentition. During my work experience at Chessington Zoo, I observed the work of the veterinary dentist and saw at first hand the differences between human and other mammals' teeth. I learnt about working with precision and speed as part of a group and using my initiative in complicated situations. While working in two dental laboratories, I gained knowledge about how dentures are prepared and the shaping and shading of porcelain crowns to look like natural teeth (ensured by communication between technician and dentist, which appealed to my artistic nature).

At school, as prefect, house official, captain of my lacrosse team and an avid member of my drama society I interacted with different age groups and learnt to organise people in a friendly but efficient manner. The interaction with people during my work experience encouraged my interest. Every other week I helped to look after an elderly lady, where I enjoy working with her team of carers. From attending a lecture at the Medical Society about diet in relation to health I was able to better understand this lady's careful diet because of her diabetes, which had led to problems with her gums and teeth due to high blood sugar levels. By reading 'Periodontal Disease – Health Policy Implications' (A Meeting on Oral Health and Systemic Health, 2002) I expanded my knowledge about the severe mouth problems that can occur from a poor diet. I continue to enjoy my visits as I like interacting with people of all ages.

I have always been intrigued by the dexterity required in dentistry. During my art A level, I completed a series of carved images from plaster, which taught me the importance of patience when working with delicate materials. I play the piano to grade 8 standard and have passed my grade 8 singing exam with distinction. Since completing my art A level, I have continued to create models with clay and enjoy painting. As House Captain of Sports and Music and through my participation in sport I have learnt the leadership and teamwork skills required to work in a team environment. As a result of my work experience, my skills and my interests I am now sure I want to study dentistry.

Example 3 shows that it is not always necessary to adhere to the three-section rule, which can become formulaic if everyone follows it. The point of a personal statement is that it should be precisely that, i.e. personal, and reflect as much as possible a candidate's individuality. Everybody is different, with different backgrounds, experiences and hobbies, and with their own individual reasons for reaching a decision to study dentistry. What should be noted in the example above is how, in each of the paragraphs, an effort has been made to link what is written as much as possible to the study of dentistry.

> **WARNING**: Do not copy any of the above passages into your personal statement, as admissions tutors are all too aware of the existence of this book. Ensure that your personal statement answer is not only personal to you, but also honest.

■ The reference

The selectors will be aware that some schools offer more in the way of activities and responsibilities than others, and they will make allowances for this. You don't have to have been on a school expedition to India, or to be head girl or head boy to be considered, but you do need to be able to demonstrate that you have taken the best possible advantage of what is on offer. The selectors will be aware of the type of school or college that you have come from (there is a section of the UCAS application that your referee fills in) and, consequently, the opportunities that are open to you. What they are looking for is that you have grasped these opportunities.

As well as your GCSE results and your personal statement, the selectors will take your reference into account. This is where your headmaster or headmistress, housemaster/housemistress or head of sixth form writes about what an outstanding person you are, how you are the life and soul of the school, how you are on target for three A grades at A level and why you will become an outstanding dentist. For him or her to say this, of course, it has to be true. The referee is expected to be as honest as possible, and to try to accurately assess your character and potential. You may believe that you have all of the qualities, academic and personal, necessary in a dentist, but unless you have demonstrated these to your teachers, they will be unable to support your application. Ideally, your efforts to impress them will have begun at the start of the sixth form (or before): you will have become involved in school activities, you will have been working hard at your studies and you will be popular with students and teachers alike. However, it is never too late, and some people mature later than others so if this does not sound like you, start to make efforts to impress the people who will contribute to your reference.

As part of the reference, your referee will need to predict the grades that you are likely to achieve. As Table 1 in Chapter 9 shows, the minimum requirement is AAB. If you are predicted lower than this, it is unlikely that you will be considered. Talk to your teachers and find out whether you are on target for these grades. If not, you need to do one or all of these:

- work harder or more effectively – and make sure that your teachers notice that you are doing so
- get some extra help either at school or outside, for instance an Easter revision course
- delay submitting your UCAS application until you have your A level results.

When to submit the UCAS application

The closing date for receipt of the application by UCAS is 15 October. Late applications are accepted by UCAS, but the dental schools are not obliged to consider them, and because of the pressure on places, it is unlikely that late applications will be considered. Although you can submit your application any time between the beginning of September and the October deadline (remembering to get it to your referee at least two weeks before the deadline so that he or she has time to prepare the reference), most admissions tutors agree that the earlier the application is submitted, the better your chance of being called for interview. Your best bet is to talk to the person who will deal with the form in the summer term of your first year of A levels, and work on your personal statement and choice of dental school over the summer holidays so that it is ready to submit at the start of the September term.

Deferred entry

Most admissions tutors are happy to consider students who take a gap year, and many encourage it. However, if you are considering a gap year, you need to make sure that you are going to use the time constructively. A year spent watching daytime TV is not going to impress anybody, whereas independent travelling, charity or voluntary work either at home or abroad, work experience or a responsible job will all indicate that you have used the time to develop independence and maturity. Above all, make sure that whatever you do with the year involves regular contact with other people.

You can either apply for deferred entry when you submit your UCAS application, in which case you need to outline your plans in your personal statement, or apply in September following the publication of your A level results. If you expect to be predicted the right grades, and the feedback from your school or college is that you will be given a good reference, you should apply for deferred entry, but if you are advised by your referee that you are unlikely to be considered, you should give yourself more time to work on your referees by waiting until you have your A level results.

What happens next?

About a week after UCAS receives your application, it will send you a welcome letter listing all of your choices. Check this carefully – make sure that the universities and courses are correct (a common mistake is to select the foundation year – the 'pre-dental' year – rather than the start of the course proper), and that your name and address are also correct. Remember also to inform UCAS if your address changes.

The next correspondence you will receive, if you are lucky, is likely to be from the dental schools, asking you to attend an interview.

You can also keep track of offers or rejections by using the online facility on the UCAS website. You will be given a password by UCAS to access this. Do not be alarmed if you do not hear anything soon after UCAS has sent you your welcome letter. Some dental schools interview on a first come, first served basis while others wait until all applications are in before deciding whom to interview. It is not uncommon for students to hear nothing until after Christmas.

If you are unlucky, you will receive a notification from UCAS telling you that you have been rejected by one or more of the dental schools. Don't despair: you may hear better news from another of the schools that you applied to. Even if you get four rejections, the worst thing that you can do is to give up and decide that it is no longer worth working hard. On the contrary, if this does happen, you should become even more determined to gain high grades so that you can apply the following year.

Note: Going through Clearing in August is no longer an option. As there are a limited number of places offered these are often oversubscribed by the greater numbers of offers made over places available. The exception to the rule in 2008 was Cardiff, which allowed only four students via Clearing. See Table 2, Chapter 9.

Checklist

- Two weeks' work shadowing?
- Right GCSEs?
- On target for AAB?
- Looked at all dental schools' prospectuses?
- Been to open days?
- Registered for the UKCAT?
- Maximum four choices on UCAS application?
- Does the personal statement demonstrate commitment, research, personal qualities, communication skills and manual dexterity?

Dental timeline

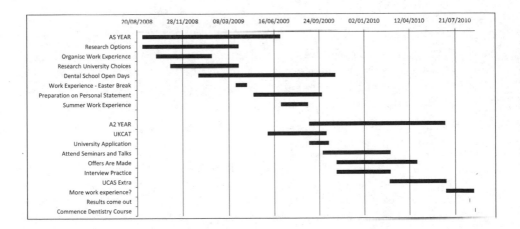

The figure shows the tasks that you will need to be aware of over a period of two years. That is, from your AS year to the end of your A2

year. This generic timeline gives an overview of the timing of some of the various tasks that you should plan for, if you are to maximise your chances of gaining entry into a dental school.

As you can see in the figure, in your lower sixth year you need to mainly start researching your courses and options, preparing the personal statement and organising work experience, at least for the AS summer break. In the second year you must hit the ground running as UKCAT preparation and UCAS applications must be completed by mid October or so. Meanwhile, in the rest of the year you could be fine tuning your interview skills ready for that call up, getting more work experience and of course studying as hard as you can, to achieve those all-important A grades. Finally, the results which come out in the third week of August will signal if you have been successful or not, as the case may be.

04 The interview stage and getting an offer

If the selectors like the picture that the UCAS application has painted of you, they will call you for interview. The purpose of the interview is to allow them to see whether this picture is an accurate one, and to investigate whether you have a genuine interest in dentistry. The interviewers will generally ask you questions designed to:

- relax you – so that they can assess your communication skills
- investigate your interest and suitability for dentistry
- get a clearer picture of your personal qualities.

Questions to get you relaxed

Question: *How was your journey here today?*
Comment: The interviewers are not really interested in the details of your journey. Do not be tempted to give them a minute-by-minute account of your bus journey ('and then we waited for six minutes at the road works on Corporation Street . . .') or to simply say 'OK'. Say something like 'It was fine, thank you. The train journey took about two hours, which gave me the chance to catch up on some reading.' With a bit of luck, they will ask you what you read, which gives you the chance to talk about a book, newspaper article or an item in *New Scientist*.

Question: *Tell me why you decided to apply to Melchester.*
Comment: Another variation on this might be 'How did you narrow your choice down to four dental schools?' The panel will be looking for evidence of research, and that your reasons are based on informed judgement. Probably the best possible answer would start with 'I came to your open day . . .' because you can then proceed to tell them why you like their university so much, what impressed you about the course and facilities and how the atmosphere of the place would particularly suit you.

If you are/were unable to attend open days, try to arrange a formal or informal visit before you are interviewed so that you can show that you are aware of the environment, both academic and physical, and that you like the place. If you know people who are at the dental school or university, so much the better. You should also know about the course structure: the prospectus will give detailed information. Given the choice between a candidate who is not only going to make a good dentist, but clearly wants to come to their institution, and another who may have the right qualities but does not seem to care whether it is there or somewhere else that he or she studies, who do you think the selectors will choose?

Answers to avoid are ones such as 'Reputation' (unless you know in detail the areas for which the dental school is highly regarded), 'It is in London, and I don't want to move away from my friends', 'You take a lot of re-take students' or 'My dad says it is easy to get a place here'.

> **WARNING**: Do your homework by reading the prospectus and looking at the website. Although on the surface all dental courses appear to cover broadly the same subjects, there are big differences between the ways courses are delivered, and in the opportunities for patient contact, and your interviewers will expect you to know about their course.

A good answer could be 'I came to an open day last summer, which is why I have applied here. I enjoyed the day, and was impressed by the facilities, and by the comments of the students who showed us around, because they seemed so enthusiastic about the course. Also, my cousin studied English at the university and I visited her, and got to sample the atmosphere of the town.' There are variations on this question. The interviewers may ask you what you know about the course, or about the dental school. In all cases, this is your chance to show the interviewers that you are desperate to come to their dental school.

Questions about dentistry

Question: *Why do you want to be a dentist?*
Comment: The question that all interviewees expect. Given that the interviewers will be aware that you are expecting the question, they will also expect your answer to be carefully planned. If you look surprised, and say something like 'Um . . . well . . . I haven't really thought about why . . .' you can expect to be rejected. Other answers to avoid are those along the lines of 'The money', 'I couldn't get into medicine', 'I want to help people' or 'I like inflicting pain'.

Many students are worried that they will sound insincere when they answer this question. The way to avoid this is to try to bring in reasons that are personal to you, for instance, an incident that started your interest (perhaps a visit to your own dentist), or an aspect of your work experience that particularly fascinated you. The important thing is to try to express clearly what interested you, rather than generalise your answers. Rather than saying 'dentistry combines science, working with people and the chance to have control over your career' – which says little about you – tell the interviewers about the way that your interest progressed. Here is an example of a good answer:

Although it seemed strange to my friends, I used to enjoy going to the dentist when I was young. This was because my dentist explained things very clearly and patiently, and I was interested in what was happening around me. When I was thinking about my career, I arranged to shadow another dentist, and the more time I spent at the surgery, the more I realised that this would really suit me. This also gave me the chance to find out about what being a dentist is really like. The things about dentistry that I particularly enjoy are . . .

WARNING: Do not learn the quote and repeat it at your interview. Ensure that your answer is not only personal to you, but also honest. With luck, the interviewers will pick up on something that you said about work experience, and ask you more questions about this. Since 'Why do you want to be a dentist?' is such an obvious question, interviewers often try to find out the information in different ways. Expect questions such as 'When did your interest in dentistry start?', or 'What was it about your work experience that finally convinced you that dentistry was for you?'

Question: *I see that you spent two weeks with your dentist. Was there anything that surprised you?*

Comment: Variations on this question could include 'Was there anything that particularly interested you?', 'Was there anything you found off-putting?' or simply 'Tell me about your work experience'. What these questions really mean is 'Are you able to show us that you were interested in what was happening during your work experience?' Returning to the original question, answering either 'Yes' or 'No' without explanation will not gain you many marks. Similarly, saying 'Yes, I was surprised by the number of patients who seemed very scared' says nothing about your awareness of the dentist's approach to his or her patients. However, answering 'Yes, I was surprised by the number of patients who seemed very scared. What struck me, however, was the way in which the dentist dealt with each patient as an individual, sometimes being sympathetic, sometimes explaining things in great detail and sometimes using humour to relax them. For instance . . .' shows that you were interested enough to be aware of more than the most obvious things.

Sentences that start with 'For example . . .' and 'For instance . . .' are particularly important as they allow you to demonstrate your interest. In order to be able to give examples, you should keep a diary of things that you saw during your work experience so that you do not forget. You should revise from this before your interview, as if you were revising for an examination.

Question: *I see that you try to keep up to date with developments in dentistry. Can you tell me about something that you have read about recently?*

Comment: If you are interested in making dentistry your career, the selectors will expect you to be interested enough in the subject to want to read about it. Good sources of information are *New Scientist*, the BDA website (www.bda.org) and national newspapers. You should get into the habit of looking at a broadsheet newspaper every day to see if there are any dentistry-related stories. Note that the question uses the word 'recently': recent does not mean an article you read two years ago – keep up to date. You could, for instance, say 'There was a recent article in *New Scientist*, about the different types of bacteria present in the mouth, only a few of which are responsible for tooth decay. At present, anti-bacterial toothpastes and mouthwashes kill all bacteria, including ones that play a beneficial role. Scientists are now working on anti-bacterials that only target specific, harmful bacteria.'

Question: *During your work experience, you had the chance to discuss dentistry with the practitioner. What do you know about the way NHS dentists are paid?*

Comment: You must be aware of the nuts and bolts of running a dental practice. You should be aware that, while NHS general practitioners are paid according to a capitation scheme (by the number of patients on their books), NHS dental practitioners are paid on the basis of the treatment that they perform. You should also have an idea about what a dentist earns and what proportion of it goes back into running the practice. Similar questions might focus on how much dentists are paid for different types of treatment, or how much NHS patients pay for treatment.

Question: *What qualities should a dentist possess?*

Comment: Don't simply list the qualities. The question has not been asked because the interviewer is puzzled about what these qualities are; it has been asked to give you a chance to show that you are aware of them, and that you possess them. The best way to answer this is to use phrases such as: 'During my work experience at the Pain-free Dental Clinic, I was able to observe/talk to the dentist, and I became aware that . . .', or 'Communication is very important. For instance, when I was shadowing my dentist, there was a patient who . . .'. Try always to relate these general questions to your own experiences.

Question: *What is the difference between tooth erosion and tooth decay?*

Comment: The interviewer is clearly not asking this question because he or she does not know the answer. The reason for the question is to find out whether you have learned about common dental problems through your discussions with dentists during work experience. As a prospective dentist, you will be expected to use technical terms more accurately than your friends who do not want to be dentists. A good answer might be: 'I asked this question to my own dentist last time I went to see her. She explained that tooth erosion is the wearing away of the tooth enamel, which can be caused by things such as fizzy drinks (which are acidic) or by grinding your teeth while you are asleep. Decay is caused by the reaction between sugar and the bacteria in plaque.'

Questions about manual dexterity

Question: *Dentistry requires a high degree of manual dexterity. Do you possess this?*

Comment: Manual dexterity means being able to perform intricate tasks with your hands. Dentists have to work in a confined and sensitive area (the mouth) using precision instruments in situations where accuracy is vital and where there is little margin for error. If you have trouble picking up a coffee cup without knocking it over, or if you always press the wrong keys when you work on a computer, dentistry may not be the best career for you. The interviewers will need reassurance that you have the manipulation skills to be able to work on other people's teeth. Good examples of tasks that require a high degree of manual dexterity include sewing, embroidery, model-making, touch-typing and playing a musical instrument. If you are not able to give an example of your own manipulative skills, take up a hobby that involves precision work now, before it is too late. Some admissions tutors like interviewees to bring in examples of their handiwork. A particularly good example of this is a student who brought in a denture that she had made during her work experience. This allowed her not only to demonstrate that she possessed the necessary skills, but also to talk about the role of the dental technician within a practice.

Case study 3: Manual dexterity

Martin Jones is a first year dental student in London. He sat A levels at a school in Birmingham, and had wanted to be a dentist since his final year of GCSEs. Martin had originally thought about pharmacy – his father is a hospital pharmacist and his mother is a nurse at another hospital – but a friend of his family, a dentist, invited him to spend a week shadowing him in his practice. Martin found the experience fascinating:

'Some of my friends had done work experience in hospitals with doctors, and they didn't really enjoy themselves. There was lots of hanging around and they were not allowed to do anything that involved patients. My time with the dentist was different. He showed me everything that was happening and let me help the nurse make fillings and take impressions. I was surprised that all of the patients agreed to let me watch what was happening. I suppose that they trusted the dentist and were happy to do what he asked.'

Martin chose Biology, Chemistry, Physics and Ceramics as his AS levels. 'To be honest, I wasn't desperately keen on Ceramics or Physics – I would have preferred English and French. However, my careers teacher thought that Ceramics might help to demonstrate manipulative skills, and the dentist that I shadowed said that Physics had helped him during his course.' He dropped Ceramics after AS with a C grade, and went on to achieve ABB in the science subjects. Martin got two interviews, one at Birmingham and the other at King's. Both concentrated heavily on his work experience. 'My advice to anyone considering dentistry is to get as much work experience as possible, and to ask questions whenever possible. Find out about everything the dentist does, and write it down at the end of the day. Funnily enough, none of the interviewers asked me about manual dexterity, so I needn't have done Ceramics – although I actually enjoyed it in the end.'

Martin's first few months studying dentistry have been hard work. 'I haven't really had a chance to relax yet – there is an enormous workload, and the social life is very hectic. I am coping because I know it is what I want to do. A couple of others on the course are having doubts because they originally wanted to do medicine.'

The question about manual dexterity is very interesting and often ignored by candidates and I would like to digress a little bit here to look at this in more detail. Manual dexterity is a very important factor which should not be overlooked in the selection process. Students, professionals and admissions tutors whom I have spoken to have all indicated that without this quality a prospective candidate might as well not continue with his or her application. Often at the interview stage students will be asked to 'Describe a situation which demonstrates your manual dexterity'. Whether at the interview stage or earlier in the personal statement, a candidate must show this clearly. So how does one demonstrate manual dexterity? The case study above indicates one way. In addition most people will talk about their hobbies, such as playing a musical instrument, or painting and drawing, design and even fixing and gluing Airfix kit models. One student I spoke to demonstrated this in the interview by showing a series of photos which showed him dismantling and building a computer.

WARNING: Do not lie about the example of manual dexterity that you describe. One admissions tutor tells the story of a boy who claimed that he liked icing cakes in his spare time. He brought in photographs of some of the cakes he had iced, but it became clear, after very little questioning, that it was his mother who had actually done the work. This did not go down well with the panel, as you can imagine!

Questions to find out what sort of person you are

Question: *What do you do to relax?*
Comment: Don't say 'Watch TV' or 'Go to the pub'. Mention something that involves working or communicating with others, for instance sport or music. Use the question to demonstrate that you possess the qualities required in a dentist. However, don't make your answer so insincere that the interviewers realise that you are trying to impress them. Saying 'I relax most effectively when I go to the local dental surgery to shadow the dentist' will not convince them.

Question: *How do you cope with stress?*
Comment: Dentistry can be a stressful occupation. Dentists have to deal with difficult people, those who are scared and those who react badly when in a dental surgery. Furthermore, there are few 'standard' situations: everyone's mouth and teeth are different, as are their problems, and things can go wrong. In these circumstances, the dentist cannot panic, but must remain calm and rational. In addition, the nature of the profession means that dentists must always be aware of the financial aspects of running a business. The interviewers will want to make a judgement as to whether you will be able to cope with the demands of the job.

Having been through it themselves, it is unlikely that they will regard school examinations as being particularly stressful. Hard work, yes, but not as stressful as training to be a dentist or practising as a dentist. What they are looking for are answers that demonstrate your calmness and composure when dealing with others. You could relate it to your work experience, or your Saturday job.

Dealing with a queue of angry and impatient customers demanding to know why their cheeseburgers are not ready can be difficult. Other areas that can provide evidence of stress management are school expeditions, public speaking, or positions of responsibility at school or outside.

Question: *I see that you enjoy reading. What is the most recent book that you have read?*
Comment: The question might be about the cinema or theatre, but the point of it is the same: to get you talking about something that interests you. Although it may sound obvious, if you have written that you enjoy reading on your UCAS application, make sure that you have actually read something recently. Admissions tutors will be able to tell you stories about interviewees who look at them with absolute surprise when they are asked about books, despite it featuring in the personal statement. Answers such as 'Well . . . I haven't had much time recently, but . . . let me see . . . I read *Elle* last month, and . . . oh yes . . . I had to read *Jane Eyre* for my English GCSE' will not help your chances. By all means put down that you like reading, but make sure that you have read an interesting novel in the period leading up to the interview, and be prepared to discuss it.

How to succeed in the interview

You should prepare for an interview as if you are preparing for an examination. This involves revision of your work experience diary so that you can recount details of your time with a dentist, revision of the newspaper, website and *New Scientist* articles that you have saved, and revision of all the things that you have mentioned on your personal statement. When you are preparing for your A levels you sit a mock examination so that the real thing does not come as a total surprise; when you are preparing for an interview, have a mock interview so that you can get some feedback on your answers. Your school may be able to help you. If not, independent sixth-form colleges usually provide a mock interview service. Friends of your parents may also be able to help. There is a list of practice interview questions below.

Mock interview questions

- Why do you want to be a dentist?
- What have you done to investigate dentistry?
- Why does dentistry interest you more than medicine?
- What are the ideal qualities that a dentist should possess?
- Do you possess these qualities?
- Give me an example of how you cope with stress.
- Why did you apply to this dental school?
- Did you come to our open day?
- During your work experience, did anything surprise you?
- During your work experience, did anything shock you?
- Is your own dentist good at communicating with his patients?
- Tell me about preventive dentistry.
- What is orthodontics?
- Why do dentists recommend the fluoridation of water supplies?
- What are the arguments against fluoridation of water supplies?
- What are amalgam fillings made of?
- What are white fillings made of?
- There has been a good deal of negative publicity about mercury fillings. Do you think that they are dangerous?
- If you had to organise a campaign to improve dental health, how would you go about it?
- What is gingivitis?
- How are NHS dentists funded? Is it the same for GPs?
- Should dental treatment be free on the NHS?
- How much does an average dentist earn?
- Have you read any articles about dentistry recently?
- What advances can we expect in dental technology/treatment in the future?
- What have you done to demonstrate your commitment to the community?

- What would you contribute to this dental school?
- What are your best/worst qualities?
- What was the last novel that you read? Did you like it?
- What was the last play/film that you saw? Did you like it?
- What do you do to relax?
- What is your favourite A level subject?
- What grades do you expect to gain in your A levels?
- Do dentists treat children differently from adults?
- What precautions need to be taken with patients who are HIV positive?
- What is an overbite?
- What do you know about forensic dentistry?
- What is the role of the dental nurse/technician?
- How does teamwork apply to the role of a dentist?
- Did the dentists you talked to enjoy their jobs?
- What is the difference between tooth erosion and tooth decay?
- What role does a dentist have in diagnosing other medical problems?
- What do you know about the new NHS reforms for dentistry?
- What do you know about the new government contract for dentists?
- What are the reasons for the increasing use of composite fillings?
- Can you think why dentists might be concerned about the increasing use of composite fillings?

Appearance and body language are important. The impression that you create can be very influential. Remember that if the interviewers cannot picture you as a dentist in future years, they are unlikely to offer you a place.

Body language

- Maintain eye contact with the interviewers.
- Direct most of what you are saying to the person who asked you the question, but also occasionally look around at the others on the panel.
- Sit up straight, but adopt a position that you feel comfortable in.
- Don't wave your hands around too much, but don't keep them gripped together to stop them moving either. Fold them across your lap, or rest them on the arms of the chair.

Speech

- Talk slowly and clearly.
- Don't use slang.
- Avoid saying 'Erm . . .', 'You know', 'Sort of'.
- Say hello at the start of the interview, and thank the interviewer(s) and say goodbye at the end.

Dress and appearance

- Wear clothes that show that you have made an effort for the interview. You do not have to wear a business suit, but a jacket and tie (men), or a skirt and blouse (women) are appropriate.
- Make sure that you are clean and tidy.
- If appropriate, shave before the interview (but avoid using overpowering aftershave).
- Clean your nails and shoes.
- Wash your hair.
- Avoid (visible) piercings, earrings (men), jeans and trainers.
- If possible, video your mock interview so that you are aware of the way that you come across in an interview situation.

■ At the end of the interview

You may be given the opportunity to ask a question at the end. Bear in mind that the interviews are carefully timed, and that your attempts to impress the panel with 'clever' questions may do quite the opposite. The golden rule is: only ask a question if you are genuinely interested in the answer (and which, of course, you were unable to find during your careful reading of the prospectus).

Questions to avoid

- What is the structure of the first year of the course?
- Will I be able to live in a hall of residence?
- When will I first have contact with patients?

As well as being boring questions, the answers to these will be available in the prospectus. If you need to ask these questions, you would have obviously not done any serious research.

Questions you could ask

- 'I haven't studied Biology at A2 level. Do you think I should go through some biology textbooks before the start of the course?' This shows that you are keen, and that you want to make sure that you can cope with the course. It will give them a chance to talk about the extra course they offer for non-biologists.
- 'Do you think I should try to get more work experience before the start of the course?' Again, an indication of your keenness.
- 'Earlier, I couldn't answer the question you asked me on fluoridation of water supplies. What is the answer?' Something that you genuinely might want to know.
- 'How soon will you let me know if I have been successful or not?' Something you really want to know.

Remember: if in doubt, don't ask a question. End by saying 'All of my questions have been answered by the prospectus and the students who showed me around the dental school. Thank you very much for an interesting day.' Smile, shake hands (if appropriate) and say goodbye.

Structure of the interview

It is also possible for you to influence the structure of the interview in the way that you answer the questions you are asked.

The selectors will have a set of questions that they may ask, designed to assess your suitability and commitment. If you answer 'Yes' or 'No' to most questions, or reply only in monosyllables, they will fire more and more questions at you. If, however, your answers are interesting and also contain statements that interest them, they are more likely to pick up on these, and you are, effectively, directing the interview. If you are asked questions that you have prepared for, there will be less time for the interviewers to ask you questions that might be more difficult to answer. For instance, at the end of your answer to a question about work experience, you might say: 'and the dentist was able to explain the effect of new technology on dentistry . . .'.

The interviewer may then say: *I see. Can you tell me about how technology is changing dentistry?* You can then embark on an answer about new types of polymers used in fillings, for instance. At the end of your explanation, you could finish with: 'which will reduce the need for amalgam fillings that contain mercury, which some people believe have an adverse effect on a person's health.' You may then be asked about the possible problems with mercury, and so on.

Of course, this does not always work, but you would be very unlucky not to have at least one of these 'signposts' that you placed in front of them followed.

How you are selected

During the interview, the panel will be assessing you in various categories. Whether or not the interview appears to be structured, the interviewers will be following careful guidelines so that they can compare candidates from different interview sessions. Some panels adopt a conversational style, whereas others are more formal. The scoring system will vary from place to place, but in general, you will be assessed in the following categories:

- reasons for the choice of dental school
- academic ability
- motivation for dentistry

- awareness of dental issues
- personal qualities
- communication skills.

You are likely to be scored in each category, and the dental school will have a minimum mark that you will have to gain if you are to be made an offer. If you are below this score, but close to it, you may be put on an official or unofficial waiting list. If this happens, you may be considered in August, should there be places available. If you are offered a place, you will receive a letter from the dental school telling you what you need to achieve in your A levels. This is called a conditional offer. Post A level students who have achieved the necessary grades will be given unconditional offers. If you are unlucky, all you will get is a notification from UCAS saying that you have been rejected. If this happens, it is not necessarily the end of the road leading you to a career in dentistry. You may be successful in Clearing, or as a post A level applicant.

When UCAS has received replies from all of your choices, it will send you a statement of offers. You will then have about a month to make up your mind about where you want to go. If you only have one offer, you have two choices. One is to accept the choice and go to that university happy in the knowledge that you are going to study the course of your dreams; the other is to reject the choice if you have decided for whatever reason that you don't want to go to that university. If you choose to go down this route, you then have to either apply the following year or apply through what is known as UCAS Extra. This is one last, extra application chance for only **one more university**, and becomes available to students from 26 February, with the deadline and last date for the application being 6 July. You will need to check with the individual university if it is part of the UCAS Extra programme, as not all dental schools offer this additional route.

If you have more than one offer, you have to accept one as your firm choice, and may accept another (a lower offer) as your insurance choice. If the place where you really want to study makes a lower offer than one of your other choices, do not be tempted to choose the lower offer as your insurance, since you are obliged to go to the dental school that you have put as your firm choice if you achieve the grades. Even if you narrowly miss, you may still be accepted by your first choice. If you decide that you do not want to go there, once the results are issued in August you will have to withdraw from the UCAS system for that year.

If you are unsuccessful, there remains the option of studying dentistry overseas (see page 63).

05 Results day

The A level results will arrive at your school on the third Thursday in August. The dental schools will have received them a few days earlier. You must make sure that you are not away on the day the results are published. Don't wait for the school to post the results slip to you. Get your teachers to tell you the news as soon as possible. If you need to act to secure a place, you may have to do so quickly.

The dental school admissions departments are well organised and efficient, but they are staffed by human beings. If there were extenuating circumstances that could have affected your exam performance and which were brought to their notice in June, it is a good idea to ask them to review the relevant letters shortly before the exam results are published.

If you received a conditional offer and your grades equal or exceed that offer, congratulations! You can relax and wait for your chosen dental school to send you joining instructions.

Warning: you cannot assume that grades of AAC satisfy an ABB, or even BBB, offer.

What to do if you hold no offer

This section takes you through the steps you should follow if you need to use the Clearing system because you have good grades but no offer. It also explains what to do if your grades are disappointing.

Chapter 9, Table 2 shows that no one, unfortunately, gets in via the Clearing system. Most dental schools will most likely allow applicants who hold a conditional offer to slip a grade (particularly if they came across well in the interview stage) rather than dust off a reserve list of those they interviewed but did not make an offer to. Still less are they likely to consider applicants who appear out of the blue – however high their grades.

If you hold three A grades but were rejected when you applied through UCAS (i.e. you did not get an offer), you need to let the dental schools know that you are out there. The best way to do this is by fax or by email. Fax and phone numbers are listed in the UCAS Handbook. If you live nearby, you can always deliver a letter in person, talk to the office staff and hope that your application will stand out from the rest. This is where establishing prior contacts with admissions staff may pay dividends as they may remember you as having made a favourable impression and may decide to allow you in despite not achieving the grades. So it pays to get to know people and to establish a working relationship.

A sample letter/fax is given below. Don't copy it word for word!

Do not forget that your referee may be able to help you. Try to persuade him or her to ring the admissions officers on your behalf – he or she will find it easier to get through than you will. If your head teacher is unable/unwilling to ring, then he or she should, at least, send a fax or email in support of your application. It is best if both faxes/emails arrive at the dental school at the same time.

1 Melchester Road
Melchester
MC2 3EF
0123 456 7890

Miss M D Whyte
Admissions Officer
Melchester University School of Dentistry
University Road
Melchester
MC1 4GH

16 August 2007

Dear Miss Whyte

UCAS No 08-123456-7

I have just received my A level results, which were: Biology A, Chemistry A, English A. I also have an A grade in AS Art.

You may remember that I applied to Melchester but was rejected after interview/was rejected without an interview. I am still very keen to study dentistry at Melchester and hope that you will consider me for any places which may now be available.

My head teacher supports my application and is faxing you a reference. Should you wish to contact him, his details are: Mr C Harrow, tel: 0123 456 7891, fax: 0123 456 7892.

I can be contacted at the above address and could attend an interview at short notice.

Yours sincerely

L M Johnson
Lucy Johnson (Miss)

If you are applying to a dental school that did not receive your UCAS application, ask your head to fax or send a copy of the form. In general, it is best to persuade the dental school to invite you to arrange for the UCAS application to be sent.

If, despite your most strenuous efforts, you are unsuccessful, you need to consider applying again. The *other* alternative is to use the Clearing system to obtain a place on a degree course related to dentistry and hope to be accepted on the dental course after you graduate.

What to do if you hold an offer but miss the grades

If you have only narrowly missed the required grades (this includes the AAC grade case described above), it is important that you and your referee fax/email the dental school to put your case before you are rejected. Here is another sample letter.

1 Melchester Road
Melchester
MC2 3EF
0123 456 7890

Miss M D Whyte
Admissions Officer
Melchester University School of Dentistry
University Road
Melchester
MC1 4GH

16 August 2007

Dear Miss Whyte

UCAS No 08-123456-7

I have just received my A level results, which were: Chemistry A, Biology A, English C.

I hold a conditional offer from Melchester of ABB and I realise that my grades may not meet that offer. Nevertheless I am still determined to study dentistry and I hope you will be able to find a place for me this year.

May I remind you that at the time of the exams I was recovering from glandular fever. A medical certificate was sent to you in June by my head teacher. My head teacher supports my application and is faxing you a reference.

Should you wish to contact him, his details are: Mr C Harrow, tel: 0123 456 7891, fax: 0123 456 7892.

I can be contacted at the above address and could attend an interview at short notice.

Yours sincerely

L M Johnson
Lucy Johnson (Miss)

If this is unsuccessful, you need to consider re-taking your A levels and applying again later in the year (see below). The other alternative is to use the Clearing system to obtain a place on a **degree course related** to medicine and dentistry such as dental technology, which is offered by University of Wales Institute Cardiff, De Montfort University and Manchester Metropolitan University and then hope to apply to the dental course after you graduate. Remember as previously mentioned, Clearing is no longer an option.

■ Re-taking A levels

The grade requirements for re-take candidates are normally higher than for first timers (in most cases AAA). You should re-take any subject where your first result was below B and you should aim for an A grade in any subject you do re-take. It is often necessary to re-take a B grade. Take advice from the college that is preparing you for the re-take.

Most subjects allow you to re-take some or all units in January. In some cases, you might be close enough to the grade boundary to risk re-taking just one unit, but bear in mind that the more units that you re-take, the fewer extra marks you have to achieve on each in order to reach the magical figure of 480 UMS – the A grade boundary. It is also worth remembering that A2 units are harder than AS units, and so you are more likely to be able to gain the extra marks that you need by re-taking an AS unit or two than by relying on the A2 units alone.

If you simply need to improve one subject by one or two grades and can re-take the exam on the same syllabus in January, then the short re-take course (September to January) is the logical option. If, on the other hand, your grades were DDE and you need to re-take all three subjects, then you probably need to spend another year on your re-takes. You would find it almost impossible to cope with three subjects and achieve an increase of nine or 10 grades within the 17 weeks or so that are available for teaching between September and January.

Independent sixth-form colleges provide specialist advice and teaching for students considering A level re-takes. Interviews to discuss this are free and carry no obligation to enrol on a course, so it is worth taking the time to talk to their staff before you embark on A level re-takes.

◼ Re-applying to dental school

Many dental schools discourage re-take candidates (see Chapter 9, Table 1) so the whole business of applying again needs careful thought, hard work and a bit of luck.

The choice of dental schools is narrower than it was the first time round. Don't apply to the dental schools that discourage re-takers unless there are some special, extenuating circumstances to explain your disappointing grades. The following are examples of excuses which would not be regarded by admissions tutors as extenuating circumstances.

- I went skiing at Easter, and was unable to revise properly because it was too cold in the evenings for me to work.
- I left my bag on the bus the week before the exams, and all of my notes were in it, so I couldn't do any revision.
- We moved house a month before the exams, and a removal man trod on my notes, and I couldn't revise properly from them.

Some reasons are acceptable to even the most fanatical opponents of re-take candidates:

- your own illness
- the death or serious illness of a very close relative.

These are just guidelines and the only safe method of finding out if a dental school will accept you is to write and ask. A typical letter is set out below. Don't follow it word for word and do take the time to write to several dental schools before you make your final choice. The format of your letter should be:

- opening paragraph
- your exam results – set out clearly and with no omissions
- any extenuating circumstances – a brief statement
- your re-take plan – including the timescale
- a request for help and advice
- closing paragraph.

Make sure that your letter is brief, clear and well presented. You can type or word-process it, if you wish. If you have had any previous contact with the admissions staff you will be able to write 'Dear Dr Smith' and 'Yours sincerely'. Even if you go to this trouble the pressure on dental schools in the autumn is such that you may receive no more than a photocopied standard reply to the effect that, if you apply, your application will be considered. Apart from the care needed in making the choice of dental school, the rest of the application procedure is as described in the first part of this guide.

1 Melchester Road
Melchester
MC2 3EF
0123 456 7890

Miss M D Whyte
Admissions Officer
Melchester University School of Dentistry
University Road
Melchester
MC1 4GH

16 August 2007

Dear Miss Whyte

Last Year's UCAS No 08-123456-7

I am writing to ask your advice because I am about to complete my UCAS application and would very much like to apply to Melchester.

You may remember that I applied to you last year and received an offer of AAB/was rejected after interview/was rejected without an interview.

I have just received my A level results, which were: Biology B, Chemistry D, English E. I also have a B grade in AS Art

I plan to re-take Chemistry in January after a 17-week course and English over a year. If necessary, I will re-take Biology from January to June. I am confident that I can push these subjects up to AAA grades overall.

What worries me is that I have heard that some dental schools do not consider re-take candidates. I am very keen not to waste a slot on my UCAS application (or your time) by applying to schools that will reject me purely because I am re-taking.

I am very keen to come to Melchester, and would be extremely grateful for any advice that you can give me.

Yours sincerely

L M Johnson

Lucy Johnson (Miss)

06 Non-standard applications

So far, this book has been concerned with the 'standard' applicant: the UK resident who is studying at least two science subjects at A level and who is applying from school or who is re-taking immediately after disappointing A levels. Dental schools accept a small number of applicants who do not have this 'standard' background. The main non-standard categories are covered below.

■ Those who have not studied science at A level

If you decide that you would like to study dentistry after having already started on a combination of A levels that does not fit the subject requirements for entry to dental school, you can apply for the 'pre-dental course'. This is offered at five university faculties of dentistry: Bristol, Cardiff, Dundee, King's and Manchester. The course covers elements of chemistry, biology and physics and lasts one academic year.

If your pre-dental application is rejected, you will have to spend a further two years taking science A levels at a sixth-form college. Independent sixth-form colleges offer one-year A level courses and certain subjects can be covered from scratch in a single year. However, only very able students can cover A level Chemistry and Biology in a single year with good results. You should discuss your particular circumstances with the staff of a number of colleges in order to select the course that will prepare you to achieve the A level subjects you need at the grades you require.

■ Overseas students

The competition for the few places available to overseas students is fierce and you would be wise to discuss your application informally with the dental school before submitting your UCAS application. Many dental schools give preference to students who do not have adequate provision for training in their own countries. You should contact the dental schools individually for advice.

According to the UCAS entrance statistics, students applying from outside the UK are much less successful than their UK counterparts in getting offers to study dentistry. In the 2007 figures, approximately only 52 overseas students gained a place to study at British universities. By way of comparison, whereas nearly 50% of UK-based applicants gain places, the figure is less than 20% for non-UK students. Further breakdown of these figures shows that approximately 25% of non-UK/EU students gain places, and about 10% of EU students are successful. There are a number of reasons for this, and these are discussed below.

Qualifications

Many overseas students are applying with qualifications that are not equivalent to A levels or other UK qualifications, the International Baccalaureate (IB), or the Irish Leaving Certificate. These students cannot be considered unless they have done a course that leads to qualifications that are recognised as being the equivalent of A levels. The dental schools' websites will quote entrance requirements in terms of A levels, IB, Scottish Highers, the Irish Leaving Certificate and other equivalent qualifications. If you are studying for other qualifications, you will need to contact the dental schools directly to ask their advice. The UCAS website also has a link to the UK government's education qualifications website, where you can check whether your examinations are suitable. If not, you will need to think about following a one-year A level programme (studying biology, chemistry and another subject) and applying during this course. Students will also need to demonstrate proficiency in English and will be asked to have an IELTS (International English Language Testing System) score of at least 6.5. Bristol University at the moment demands an IELTS score of 7.0 (source: www.bristol.ac.ukdentalpg/buold/tuitionfees.html).

The application form

Students who are studying outside the UK are often at a disadvantage because they may not have access to the application form or lack advisers at their schools who are familiar with the requirements of a successful application. The two areas that tend to be weakest are the personal statement and the reference. Students who are unfamiliar with UCAS applications often write unsuitable personal statements, which concentrate too much on non-essential information (prizes, awards, responsibilities) and not enough on matters relevant to dentistry. It is important to explain why you wish to study dentistry in the UK rather than in your home country. Detailed advice on the personal statement can be found in Chapter 4. Similarly, your referee needs to be familiar with what the dental schools require in the reference. The UCAS website contains a section on information for referees: you should ensure that your chosen referee is familiar with this.

Work experience

Dental schools almost always require applicants to have gained some relevant work experience, and often to have done some voluntary work as well. Work experience tells the selectors that the candidates are serious about becoming dentists and that they are familiar with what the profession demands. Voluntary work demonstrates that the applicant has the caring nature necessary to work with patients. Gaining work experience can be difficult, but you should make every effort to do so. If it is impossible for you to gain dental work experience, you might try to substitute it with hospital work, or by attending relevant lectures. It is important that the reference mentions why there is a lack of work experience mentioned in the application, and what you did to try to get that experience.

In addition to gaining several weeks of work experience, there are short courses run within hospitals by dentists, giving an insight into the profession. This is particularly useful for those who are not convinced if dentistry is the right profession for them and also for those who have made up their minds but may wish to gain a further insight and have a good talking point for interview. Visit www.mdexperience.co.uk for further information on these short seminars.

Interviews

Most dental schools require students to attend interviews. This is often difficult to arrange for students who are not based in the UK. It is worth contacting the dental schools before you apply in order to see whether they would require you to travel to the UK to be interviewed.

Quotas

Whilst there is no restriction on places for EU students (who will be considered alongside UK applicants), the UK government imposes quotas for non-UK/EU students. For example, King's can only accept eight non-EU international students each year. In general, students from countries that do not have adequate training programmes for dentistry are likely to have an advantage.

If you are serious about studying dentistry in the UK, then do not be put off by the statistics. It is worth bearing in mind that whilst almost all of the UK applicants will be suitably qualified to study dentistry and will be aware of the entrance requirements (academic and other), a high proportion of overseas applicants will be rejected simply because they have not researched the requirements properly. So, careful preparation will give you a good chance of being considered. In 2007, over 60 overseas applicants were successful and many go on to have a long and fruitful career, often staying in the UK. The following case study gives such an illustration.

Case study 4: Overseas student

Saba Saied is a fourth year dental student at Barts and the London, Queen Mary's School of Medicine and Dentistry. 'I came to London to study dentistry, having studied the International Baccalaureate at an international school in Austria. I always had an interest in the sciences and knew that my career would involve them, as well as involving people and the chance to use my hands. Before starting the course, I took a year out to travel and to gain work experience, both of which helped me to gain a sense of the real world. I also learnt a great deal about myself.

'Throughout the course, I have tried to maintain a balance between work and a social life. The first two years were pre-clinical, and were spent at the Mile End campus, a friendly place full of atmosphere and students from a wide range of courses. Here we were taught the theoretical basics of medical science. The time between lectures gave us the chance for self-directed learning, and the tutorials gave us the chance to improve our understanding of the material covered in the lectures and the practicals.

'For the next three years I am at Whitechapel, where the medics and dentists are based. The dental school is buzzing all of the time, with patients of all shapes, sizes and colours. We have a great deal of responsibility, including booking our patients, calling them up and arranging appointments. I really enjoy the chance to put communication skills, psychology and sociology into practice.

'The first contact with our patients was exciting and nerve-racking. We had been well prepared and had been given the opportunity to watch and assist the students in the years above us, but now the onus was on us. You get to realise that experience is the only way to learn about clinical dentistry and dealing with patients.

'The social life is great. There is always something happening, from quiz nights to the college's clubs and societies, and although having only one year left makes me glad that I will soon be going out into the world to start working, I will miss student life enormously.

'Since starting here, I have found that dentistry is more than just a career that involves work: it is basically about patients.'

Mature students

Each year a small percentage of the entrants to dentistry are graduates, usually aged between 22 and 30 (see Chapter 9, Table 2). In exceptional circumstances, candidates who are over 30 may be considered. In general, there are two types of mature applicants:

- those who have always wanted to study dentistry but who failed to get into dental school when they applied from school in the normal way
- those who came to the idea later on in life, often having embarked on a totally different career.

The first type of mature applicant has usually followed a degree course in a subject related to medicine or dentistry, obtained a good grade (minimum 2.1) and hopes to gain some exemption from part of the pre-clinical course. These students have an uphill path into dentistry because their early failure tends to prejudice the selectors. Nevertheless, they do not have the problem of taking science A levels at a late stage in their education. If you want to follow this option you should apply through Clearing for one of the dentistry-related degrees, such as:

- anatomy
- biomedical sciences
- biochemistry
- human biology
- medical science
- pharmacology
- physiology.

The second category of mature student is often of more interest to the dental school selectors and interviewers. Applications from people aged under 30 who have achieved success in other careers and who can bring a breadth of experience to the dental school and to the profession are welcomed.

The main difficulty facing those who come late to the idea of studying dentistry is that they rarely have scientific backgrounds. They face the daunting task of studying science A levels and need very careful counselling before they embark on what will, inevitably, be quite a tough programme. Independent sixth-form colleges provide this counselling as part of their normal interview procedure.

Studying abroad

One option for those who have been unsuccessful with their applications is to study dentistry abroad – for example at Charles University in the Czech Republic or Comenius University in Bratislava, capital of Slovakia. These 5–6-year courses are taught in English and the graduate degrees are recognised by the UK's General Dental Council.

It is advisable for anyone applying for UK dental school that they have a back-up option to study dentistry in Europe, in the event that their application in the UK is unsuccessful. As applications are made via M&D Europe and not via UCAS, applicants who are offered a place to study dentistry in Europe are not obliged to accept their place if they choose to study in the UK.

Applicants who have completed up to science A level standard (or equivalent) are invited for an entrance examination, usually in April of each year in London, held by M&D Europe. Applicants who have already completed their A levels may be exempted from this examination.

The M&D Pre-Med Programme run by the University of Sussex usually confirms a place to study dentistry in European countries, if applicants are unsuccessful in securing a place at a UK dental school. Although the M&D Pre-Med is run predominantly for medical students, some UK dental schools have agreed to consider and have accepted students from this programme. See www.mdpremed.com for more details.

07 Careers in dentistry

General dental practitioners (GDPs)

According to the NHS, there were 20,850 NHS GDPs in the UK in 2008, an increase of 3.2% on 2007. Some of these dentists run their own dental practices while others work in larger practices or groups of practices. Most dental practices offer both NHS and private treatment. Private patients are offered a much wider range of treatment, but they or their dental insurance scheme providers pay the full cost, which is determined by the dentist rather than the NHS. About one million people have private dental plans.

Regardless of this, following graduation all dentists follow a similar path. During their final year at dental school, students need to consider where they wish to begin their dental career. The path chosen will vary, depending upon the individual student's abilities and interests. Many dental schools organise 'Going into Practice' days for their students, supplementing information available from the BDA.

Students qualifying at a UK dental school must complete one year of compulsory vocational training (VT) within a primary care trust (PCT) (local area) dental practice. During VT, the newly graduated dentists (known as vocational dental practitioners or VDPs) work in approved dental practices, under supervision. VDPs are paid by the NHS, and their trainers are also paid an allowance. Any earnings generated by a VDP go to the trainer. Following vocational training, dentists usually enter an established general practice as an **associate** or as an **assistant**.

There is a difference between assistant dentists and associate dentists. Assistant dentists are employed by the practice owner, and are paid a salary; associate dentists are self-employed, and responsible for the treatment that they provide, but work in a practice owned by someone else. The associate dentist buys services from the practice owner, such as nursing or technician support, materials and access to patients, by paying the practice owner either a percentage of his/her earnings, or a fixed monthly fee. In some areas, a number of practices prefer to employ **assistant** dentists. An assistantship provides an opportunity to work as a full member of the practice team but without the uncertainties of a role as an associate.

Later on, many dentists then take the step of becoming a practice owner, either becoming a partner, buying a practice or establishing a new practice. Like medical general practitioners, they have the opportunity to form long-term relationships with their patients and provide them with continuing care. This means that in addition to being dentists they are also business people, as this is what a practice is. They are now responsible not only for the treatment that they provide for their own patients, but also for the administration of the practice, and the employment of associate dentists if necessary. This is an aspect of the career that attracts many students to the profession. Thus, as well as an ability to get on well with people, it is essential to have an aptitude for business, since the dentist is a manager and team leader running a small business.

Case study 5 illustrates the experience of one dentist through the VT programme.

Case study 5: A qualified dentist

Dr Neva Patel qualified from King's six years ago: 'When I qualified, I wasn't sure whether I wanted to become a general dental practitioner (GDP), or to work in another field, such as orthodontics or paedodontics. I decided to spend a year in the hospital to gain experience in a range of dental fields.

'Working as a house officer was a very comfortable way of being introduced to dentistry – I saw four to five patients a session, and was able to call upon experts if and when the need arose. However, I did not particularly enjoy hospital politics, and I also realised that I did not want a career in research, and so I started my vocational training (VT), the compulsory year's training under a dentist in a dental practice.

'I was very lucky with my trainer, who was extremely helpful and supportive, and I enjoyed the year at the practice so much that I stayed on to practise there, and have been there ever since. Among my group of friends who qualified as dentists, I was the only one to stay on at the same practice after VT. I started off gently, seeing perhaps five to 10 patients a day, so that I could spend time on the treatment. At first, I could take up to an hour on a filling, but I soon became quicker and more confident. The big difference between now and when I first started is that I am not worried about what will come in through the door – I feel that I can cope with anything. The job does have stressful times, of course, particularly when dealing with difficult or aggressive patients. However much you are taught about stress management and dealing with anxious patients at dental school, it cannot prepare you for the real thing.

'Some patients can be aggressive because they are scared. I find that the best way to deal with nervous patients is to explain to them exactly what I am doing at all times. Whenever I use a new instrument, I tell the patient what it is for, and what I will do with it. I explain why I am taking X-rays, and the likely lifetime of the treatment that I am performing. Otherwise, they cannot see what is going on, and can become more frightened.

'The best part of the job, for me, is when my patients are genuinely pleased with the treatment: I find it very gratifying when new patients are referred by existing ones. I also like the flexibility of the job, and the fact that I can control my hours.

'My position is slightly unusual because I am a salaried dentist. This enables me to spend more time with my patients if they need it, and to devote some time to teaching patients about dental health. I don't have to worry about filling my day to maximise my earnings. It means that there is a limit to what I earn, but it also adds to job satisfaction.'

Hospital and community dentists

Hospital dentistry

Hospital dentistry concentrates on more specialist areas such as orthodontics, restorative dentistry for victims of accidents or illness, paediatric dentistry or oral medicine. As a hospital dentist, the career path is similar to that followed by a doctor: junior, specialty and so on, up to consultant level.

Unlike GDPs, hospital dentists receive a salary. Thus hospital dentistry is possibly less risky, as it is salaried full-time employment (see Case study 5 also). Hospital dentists generally work as part of a team, have access to specialised diagnostic facilities and work with consultants in other specialisations. Another advantage is that within the hospital service there is a prescribed and well-defined career structure and training pathway. However, the hours are not as flexible and time will be spent 'on call', resulting in long working sessions.

Community dental service

Some newly qualified dentists prefer to follow a more structured path, and choose to become part of the Community Dental Service (CDS), which provides dental treatment for patients with special needs, or to work in a hospital. As with the hospital service, these posts are salaried and there is a career structure, but this option is less structured than working within the hospital setting.

For further information regarding the CDS VT scheme, you should contact the various postgraduate deaneries in the UK (see Chapter 9, Table 5 for regional contact numbers and www.eastman.ucl.ac.uk/education/careerguide/index.html).

Having completed VT, experience is gained as a community clinical dental officer (CCDO) with further opportunity to gain postgraduate qualifications by part-time study. Ambitious CCDOs may wish to become senior dental officers (SDOs) with special responsibilities, e.g. for health promotion, epidemiology or treating patients with special needs (source: www.nhscareers.nhs.uk/details/Default.aspx?Id=686).

Other careers in dentistry

Dentists can also find employment in the armed services and within industry. For those with an interest in the academic aspects of dentistry, there are opportunities for research or teaching within universities. Some dentists will opt for academia and will become teachers or lecturers in dental schools, and/or involved in research.

Dentistry in the armed forces

According to the BDA, all three defence forces employ dentists to provide a comprehensive service for service personnel, both abroad and in the UK. Dentists hold a commissioned rank and there is a very structured career path. If you choose to practise in the armed forces, financial scholarships may be available during your dental studies. For more information on careers in armed forces dentistry visit the army's website and the Defence Dental Services' website, provided by the Ministry of Defence (MoD):

- www.mod.uk/DefenceInternet/AboutDefence/WhatWeDo/Health andSafety/DDS/
- www.army.mod.uk/5321.aspx

Dental bodies corporate (DBCs)

A relatively new development is the increased possibility of working for a body corporate, some of which actively recruit dentists from overseas. The BDA has an advice sheet on working for corporate bodies, which is available to members. By law, DBCs have to be registered with the General Dental Council. This area is currently on the increase due to a general move away from NHS dentistry, a growing consumerism among the general public (e.g. wealthier patients demanding top-notch care), and deregulation of the profession allowing dentists to advertise, thus making company branding possible. A further reason given by the BDA is the belief of venture capitalists, among others, that investment in dentistry will yield attractive returns.

Dentistry in industry

Some large manufacturing and engineering companies (for example oil companies and car manufacturers) offer dental services to their employees. These posts are salaried but the role is equivalent to that of a GDP.

University teaching and research

If you like both teaching and research at university level, there are opportunities in this field. Careers in university dental schools allow you to specialise in a particular aspect of dentistry, which can enable you to pursue a particular interest in greater depth. University dental teachers will have gained postgraduate qualifications and can progress to become senior lecturers or professors and, if they so wish, get involved in writing teaching materials.

Running a business

A dental practice is a business which rents/buys a site, employs qualified staff, trains staff, pays business tax and so on. The income of a practice serves to pay the employees, rates and rent. A proportion of the profit is reinvested in the practice for new equipment or new facilities, so that the practice may continue to offer the best service to the patients. Dentists will be managing a team of people encompassing dental nurses, hygienists, receptionists and others, so good administrative and managerial abilities are needed. While practices can often be very successful and lucrative, drawbacks must not be under rated, including long hours, stress, difficult patients or staff and frustrations with the NHS. These are all elements that a dentist can find disheartening and unpleasant.

Dental nurses

Perhaps the most important person as far as the dentist is concerned is the dental nurse, who plays a key role in any dental practice. Working alongside the dentist, it is the nurse's job to provide a high standard of care for patients and to be the dentist's assistant. They provide skilled supportive care and are able to perform diagnostic tests such as X-rays.

Dental hygienist

The dental hygienist also is a very important part of the dental team. He or she is a licensed dental professional with a degree or diploma who specialises in preventive dental care, focusing on techniques in oral hygiene. In most cases, the hygienist is employed by a dental practice. Procedures performed by hygienists include cleaning, scaling, radiography and dental sealing.

Receptionists

The first person you will encounter when you telephone or visit a dental practice is the receptionist(s). The receptionist is there to effectively manage the bookings of patients wishing to see the dentist. In practices where there are multiple practitioners, efficient and effective receptionists and administration staff are crucial to the viability and long-term profit and health of the practice. In taking care of the appointments process and correspondence details of a busy practice, they allow dentists more time to focus on their work.

The point of mentioning the above two roles here is to make you aware of some of the important people that you will need to find, train and keep – another aspect of running a business.

Case study 6: Private practice

Stephen Fenny has been a practice owner, working in London, for 15 years. 'What I get out of being a dentist is working with the people that I treat, not the mechanics of the job. The job is repetitive and often stressful, particularly as I run my own business and have to be aware of the balance between providing the best possible treatment for my patients and the economics of running the practice. Today, I saw 29 patients – slightly more than usual because of school half-term – and I need to ensure that I juggle my time effectively, so that an unexpected problem with one patient does not cause delays for others. Being reassuring and comforting throughout the day, whilst trying to deal with a large number of patients, brings about its own form of stress. Having said that, for me, people are the excitement of the job, and the thing that makes being a dentist enjoyable and worthwhile.'

■ Women in the professions

It was little over a century ago that Lilian Murray (later Lindsay) became the first qualified woman dentist in 1895. In 2007, 37% of practising dentists in the UK were women. According to the BDA, by the year 2020 this figure is expected to rise to over 50%. Today more than 50% of new entrants to dental undergraduate courses in the UK are female. Therefore, in just over a century, women have gone from not being represented in the profession to acceptance and potential dominance.

Dentistry is a good career choice for a woman and, according to a BDA survey, 93% of women dentists responded that their positive career expectations when entering dental school had been fulfilled. Women leaving dental school expect that, if they wish, they will be able to combine a professional career with caring for a family and/or undertaking postgraduate study. Thus, the primary reasons in the survey appeared to be career flexibility, caring and working with people and the opportunity to combine practical and intellectual work. Anticipated financial rewards did not seem to be a major factor.

Case study 7: Combination of career and family

Sarah sat her A levels in Biology, Chemistry and Maths in a school in Kent, and gained grades ABB, respectively. She chose King's from the three dental schools that offered her a place, because she wanted to study in London. She says, 'I enjoyed studying alongside the doctors, as they tended to be a bit more lively than the dentists. I think that they need to get it out of their systems, because when they qualify, they have very little time for a personal life, whereas being a dentist gives you more flexibility to separate work from social life.'

Sarah now works in Sussex, as an associate dentist in a practice in a small town. 'I like the fact that many of my patients live in the country, and are more interested in keeping their teeth healthy than in cosmetic dentistry – in cities, people tend to be more vain.'

Her advice for women thinking of dentistry as a career: 'You need to be physically quite strong, because you are on your feet a lot of the time, and performing extractions is hard work. In many ways it is an advantage being a woman, because children are less intimidated by you. What do I dislike about being a dentist? The way that people react when you tell them what you do – they always have a horror story to tell about their dentists when they were children. The best thing? I will be able to continue my career when I have children.'

Salaries and wages

According to Prospects Planner (www.prospectus.ac.uk) a typical starting salary for a first year out dentist as a VDP is £28,600 – this was the case in January 2008. This wage on average is expected to rise after 10–15 years anywhere between £60,000 and £141,000. This large disparity depends on whether a dentist chooses to stay and work within the NHS system (in a PCT) or in the CDS. On average, dentists working for the CDS can expect to earn between £36,000 and £77,000.

It is not surprising that in the private sector dentists will learn around the £120,000 to £140,000 mark after expenses. This can, of course, be far greater, depending on the type of dental practice and the amount of work a dentist is prepared to do. For instance surgical and cosmetic dentistry are two areas which command the high-end costs of the market. A salaried consultant for the NHS can earn up to £160,000. Consultants work short contracts, six to 12 months, irregular hours and have on-call responsibilities.

08 Current issues/ topics

Fluoridation

What is fluoride?

Fluorine is a naturally occurring gas. When fluorine forms a binary compound with another element, this compound is known as a fluoride. Fluoride ions are found in soil, fresh water and seawater, plants and many foods. It has a beneficial effect on dental health.

How does fluoride work?

Fluoride is beneficial to both developing and developed teeth as it decreases the risk of decay. Dental decay is caused by acids produced by the plaque on our teeth, which react with the sugars and other carbohydrates we eat. The acids attack the tooth enamel which, after repeated attacks, will break down, allowing cavities to form. Fluoride acts by bonding to the tooth enamel and reducing the solubility of the enamel in the acids. Fluoride also inhibits the growth of the bacteria responsible for tooth decay. There is also evidence that it helps repair the very earliest stages of decay by promoting the remineralisation of the tooth enamel. Fluoride is not a cure-all and the risk of tooth decay can still be increased by other factors such as exposed roots, frequent sugar and carbohydrate consumption, poor oral hygiene and reduced salivary flow.

How was fluoride discovered to be beneficial to dental health?

The earliest work on the benefits of fluoridation was the studies of Frederick MacKay, a dentist in Colorado in the early 1900s. MacKay noted a condition in his patients which was previously not described in the literature. Many of his patients had a strange brown staining on their teeth. Subsequent research by MacKay and a colleague, D V Black, resulted in the discovery that mottled enamel (what we now refer to as dental fluorosis) was due to imperfections in the formation of the tooth enamel. They also noticed that individuals with dental fluorosis had teeth that were particularly resistant to decay. MacKay continued his research and discovered the link between dental fluorosis and the naturally high levels of fluoride in the drinking water in Colorado Springs.

What is fluoridation?

Fluoride occurs naturally in our water supply. Fluoridation is the process by which the amount of fluoride is adjusted to the optimum level that protects against tooth decay. The optimum level is one part per million (ppm). With a few exceptions, levels in UK water supplies are considerably lower than the optimum value.

What are the benefits of fluoridation?

Initially the main beneficiaries of fluoridated water supplies were thought to be children under the age of five years. In areas where the concentration of fluoride in water supplies is 1 ppm, rates of decay and tooth loss in children are greatly reduced. High levels of tooth decay in children are generally associated with areas of social deprivation. This is a pattern repeated throughout the EU and the USA. The best dental health regions in the UK are the West Midlands, an area where over two-thirds of the population receive fluoridated water, and South East England, which is predominantly an affluent area. The worst areas for dental health are those associated with high levels of social deprivation, such as North West England and Scotland. Children living in socially deprived areas with non-fluoridated water supplies can have up to six times more tooth decay than those living in more affluent areas or those receiving fluoridated water supplies. For example, in the poorest communities of North West England as many as one in three children of pre-school age have had a general anaesthetic for tooth extraction, and in Glasgow tooth extraction is the most common reason for general anaesthesia for children under the age of 10.

Subsequent research has shown that it is not only children who benefit from fluoridated water supplies but people of all ages, as the effect of fluoride on the surface of fully developed teeth is thought to be even more important. Elderly people, in particular, can benefit from drinking fluoridated water. The decrease in salivary flow with age, combined with reduced manual dexterity, means it is more difficult to keep your teeth clean as you get older. So older people are more prone to root surface decay, which is difficult to treat. As fluoride strengthens adult tooth enamel it helps reduce the incidence of this type of decay.

Probably the two most important advantages of fluoridated water supplies as opposed to any other method of combating tooth decay are that it is cost-effective and, most importantly, that all members of the community are reached, regardless of income, education or access to dental care.

What are the problems with fluoridation?

One of the side effects of an excessive intake of fluoride is dental fluorosis. This is mottling of the teeth caused by a disruption of the enamel formation while the teeth are developing under the gums. It occurs between birth and the age of five years, when the enamel is developing. In mild cases dental fluorosis is purely a minor cosmetic problem, which is barely visible to either the individual or the observer. It is also thought that mild dental fluorosis may further increase the resistance of the tooth enamel to decay. In moderate to severe cases of dental fluorosis, the colouring of the teeth is very pronounced and irregularities develop on the tooth surface. Whether this is purely a cosmetic problem or whether it adversely affects the function of the teeth is a matter of some debate.

Some research has claimed links between fluorosis and higher instances of bone cancer, osteoarthritis and fractures. At present scientific studies supporting these findings are rare and they remain somewhat unsubstantiated, with the majority of scientific opinion believing there to be no link between fluoridated water supplies and these diseases. The reasons for the varying rates of tooth decay and loss in children are complex but include the amount of sugar in their diet, the availability, affordability and use of fluoride toothpaste and the presence of fluoride in other areas of their diet, e.g. water, milk and salt. Fluoridation of water supplies does not tackle the underlying issue of educating people in good oral hygiene and better diet.

Other concerns expressed about fluoridation are its effect on the environment, particularly on plants. Fluorides have been used in some pesticides and insecticides and their use is now restricted. Other industrial fluorides are one of the main pollutants in lakes, rivers, streams and the atmosphere.

What are the ethical issues involved in fluoridation?

One of the main ethical issues with fluoridation of water supplies involves infringement of personal liberty, as it effectively medicates everyone without an individual having the choice to refuse. We have no choice of water supply other than what is supplied through our water company, unless we opt to buy bottled water, the cost of which would be prohibitive for certain sections of the community.

The other main issue is whether one segment of society should benefit while another is potentially put at risk. By giving fluoridated water supplies to individuals who have a high intake of fluoride from other sources, they could theoretically be put at risk – but by an action that would, according to present scientific opinion, benefit thousands of deprived children.

What is the situation in the UK?

In the UK less than 10% of water supplies are fluoridated. Approximately 5.5 million people, mainly in the West Midlands and North East

England, receive optimally fluoridated water. At present in the UK, water companies can block fluoridation schemes despite health authorities' wishes. The government is intending to change the law so that water companies have to comply with the wishes of the local health authority. However, fluoridation would only be introduced following extensive publicity and public consultation.

The areas in most need of fluoridated water supplies are those with high tooth decay rates, including Merseyside and other parts of North West England, Yorkshire, Scotland, Wales and Northern Ireland, plus some socially deprived communities in the South, such as Inner London.

Who supports water fluoridation in the UK?

- British Dental Association
- British Medical Association
- British Fluoridation Society
- World Health Organization

What is the situation in other parts of the world?

The pattern of socially deprived areas having a high incidence of tooth decay is repeated throughout the EU. Policy throughout the EU varies, with some member states having optimally fluoridated water supplies. Others support the idea but for various reasons do not have fluoridated supplies (e.g. Sweden and the Netherlands). The other main recipients of fluoridated water are the USA (60%) and Australia (above 65%).

What other products have fluoride added?

Several other methods of increasing fluoride intake have been used, the most obvious of which is toothpaste. Salt fluoridation has been used as an alternative to water fluoridation in several countries, including Switzerland, France, Belgium, Colombia, Jamaica and Costa Rica. This has the advantage of not requiring a centralised piped water system. However, it is not without its problems: dosage must take into account the other sources of fluoride in the area, ensuring intake is not excessive. The production of fluoridated salt also requires specialist technology. Another consideration is the link between consumption of sodium and hypertension, which would make this method of fluoride intake unsuitable for some individuals.

Experiments using fluoridated milk supplies have also been carried out. So far these have been small studies in which fluoride is added to milk given to children in nursery and primary schools (tests have been carried out in Bulgaria, Russia and the UK). This would directly target children. However, absorption of fluoride from milk is thought to be slower than from water. Another problem would be monitoring and controlling fluoride administered in this manner, as it would be more difficult than with water because of the number of dairies involved. Fluoridated milk would also have to have an adjusted dosage of fluoride, depending on whether the water supply was already naturally fluoridated or not. Additionally, a significant number of people do not drink milk for health or other reasons.

Mercury fillings

Amalgam fillings (often known as 'silver' fillings) – the most common type of metal fillings – contain a high proportion (about 50%) of mercury, a toxic metal. The remainder is made up of copper, tin, silver and zinc. There has always been a belief that the mercury could not escape from the mixture, but there is some evidence that mercury vapour does escape. The BDA accepts that a tiny amount may escape, but that this amount is harmless to most (97%) of the population. Some countries have banned the use of mercury in fillings, among them Sweden and Austria. Critics of mercury in fillings claim that the mercury vapour can cause gum disease, kidney, liver and lung problems, Alzheimer's disease and multiple sclerosis. The British Society for Mercury-free Dentistry recommends the removal of amalgam fillings, to be replaced by composite fillings, but only if precautions are taken to ensure that mercury is not ingested or inhaled. 'White' fillings – made of composite materials or polymers – can be used in place of silver fillings, but they are not as strong and so can often be unsuitable for the back teeth, which are subjected to greater stress than the front teeth. Also being developed is the 'smart filling' – a filling that releases calcium and phosphate ions on contact with acids from the tooth bacteria that cause decay. These ions not only stop the decay, but also help to repair damage.

Was my treatment necessary?

It is clear that, since dentists are paid for the treatment that they perform, the more treatment, or the more complex the treatment is, the more the dentist will earn. While the great majority of dentists are scrupulous about providing only appropriate treatment, there have been well-publicised cases of dentists providing unnecessary fillings, crowns or extractions, simply to make more money. The *Guardian*, in an article 'Do dentists put the bite on patients?' (May 1999), carried out an experiment (albeit limited) to test this: a reporter booked examinations at a number of surgeries in London, and the recommendations ranged from one filling and a trip to the hygienist (cost £32.92 then) to two fillings and three replacement crowns (£915 then). Even bearing in mind that dentists have to use their professional judgement as to whether treatment is urgently required, or whether it could be delayed, the range of recommended treatment in this particular instance is staggering. The

BDA commented on the survey by saying 'Differences in diagnosis are not unusual. It is a matter of judgement and opinion and much will depend on what the patient wants. If you saw lots of GPs you would probably obtain lots of different diagnoses as well.'

The BDA website has some useful information on the reasons why dentists sometimes disagree on the nature or the extent of treatment. Dental decay often progresses slowly and the point at which treatment becomes necessary is a matter of judgement. When a dentist decides that treatment is appropriate, there is often more than one type of treatment that is appropriate. According to the BDA:

> 'A dentist's advice about treatment will depend on a number of factors – whether the patient has been seen before, a dentist's understanding of a particular problem the patient might have, the patient's oral hygiene (which might make certain advanced forms of treatment less feasible), the patient's timescale, and so on.'

The new NHS reforms aim to reduce the amount of unnecessary treatment. The NHS undertakes checks to ensure that patients are getting appropriate treatment by asking a sample of the patients from each NHS dentist in the UK to attend a check-up by an independent dentist to assess the amount and the quality of the treatment.

The nation's teeth

There has been a steady improvement in dental health in the UK. According to the very comprehensive report by the Office of Population Censuses and Surveys, in 1978, 30% of the adult population had lost all of their natural teeth, but by 1998 this figure had fallen to 13%. In 1998, adults who still had their own teeth had, on average, 15.8 sound and untreated teeth, compared with 13.0 in 1978. The average number of missing teeth fell from 9.0 in 1978 to 7.2 in 1998. The average number of decayed teeth also fell from 1.9 to 1.0. The next survey is due in 2009 (this survey is done every 10 years). Reasons for the improvement include:

- fluoridation of water
- fluoride in toothpaste
- developments in dental treatment
- provision of preventive and restorative dental treatment
- increased awareness of dental health.

In 2003, a survey into the health of children's teeth revealed that although the health of children's teeth is continuing to improve, there is a big gap between the best and the worst, and some of this is to do with regional differences (www.statistics.gov.uk/children/dentalhealth). Professor Liz Kay, Scientific Adviser to the BDA (quoted on the BDA's website), said:

> 'While this report does demonstrate a welcome overall improvement in children's dental health, the gulf between those with the best and worst oral health persists. This report shows that a high percentage of our children still suffer unacceptable levels of tooth decay.'

A report in the March 2004 edition of the *British Dental Journal* says that children from Asian backgrounds have healthier teeth. According to the report, over 60% of white children have some tooth erosion, compared with under 50% of children from Asian families. In both groups, boys were more likely to be affected than girls. The report highlights the statistical correlation between high levels of sugar in the diet and levels of tooth erosion. Different dietary habits between the two groups, therefore, might be part of the explanation.

One of the major contributing factors towards tooth decay and erosion in children is the consumption of fizzy drinks. According to the BDA, the effect of consuming any fizzy drink increases the chance of tooth erosion in 14-year-olds by 220% (and over 90% of 14-year-olds drink fizzy drinks). Children who drink several fizzy drinks a day have a 500% increase in the chance of damage occurring to their teeth.

The National Institute for Health and Clinical Excellence (NICE) has published new guidelines on the recommended frequency of dental check-ups. The recommended interval between check-ups has been the same (usually six months) regardless of the patient's age and oral health, but Ralph Davies of the BDA, quoted on the BDA's website, said:

> 'The British Dental Association has always held that the frequency of dental check-ups should be based on the individual patient, not a "one size fits all" system. How often you need an examination should be based on what is best for you as a patient and the clinical judgement of your dentist. NICE has also called for more research to be carried out on this subject and the BDA strongly supports this.'

The new guidelines might also help to cut the waiting lists for NHS dentists. It has been estimated that the NHS is nearly 2,000 dentists short of what is needed to provide an effective oral care system in England. This shortage is predicted to rise to over 5,000 by 2011, according to *The Times* (October 2004). Less than 50% of adults in England have attended an NHS dentist. The government has agreed to spend over £350 million on NHS dentistry reforms and on the recruitment of 1,000 new dentists.

Fillings could be history

Over the past 30 years, our teeth have got much better. We look after them better, visit the dentist more and are more 'tooth aware'. It is now common for people over the age of 30 to boast that they have never had a filling or crown – something unheard of a generation ago. However, many people still get cavities and so drilling and filling have not gone away. Now a new treatment promises an end to this as well. It is not yet widely available (a handful of private dental practices across the country use the treatment) but HealOzone could, according to its supporters, banish unsightly fillings once and for all from our mouths. The treatment involves using a laser to detect tooth decay. Then the tooth is enclosed in a special airtight rubber cup and the air removed and replaced by ozone, a powerful germicide. The ozone instantly kills the bacteria that cause decay and the cavity in the tooth either 'remineralises' naturally, aided by calcium salts in our saliva, or if the hole is too big, is filled with a cosmetic white filling without the need for drilling. Remineralisation is aided by a mouthwash containing fluoride, calcium, zinc, phosphate and xylitol.

A spokesman for James Hull Associates (JHA), one of the largest chains of dental practices to offer HealOzone, reported that 'It works in 90% of cases at the first treatment. It takes 40 seconds a tooth against the half-hour process of injections, drilling and filling. Once the equipment has been purchased (about £15,000) the treatments could also prove to be cheaper than the more conventional treatments.'

The BDA, while being impressed with some of the early results, has asked for the use of ozone in the medical field to be monitored carefully.

> 'It is not new, its use in the medical field extends back to before the First World War and some countries (for example Cuba) still use it very extensively. Whilst it is very useful in the upper atmosphere it is a pollutant and a major cause of smog and respiratory problems.'

JHA countered by saying that each tooth is isolated within an airtight rubber cup and the treatment is so localised that there is not a problem. The Federal Food and Drug Administration (FDA) in the USA is adamant that:

> 'ozone is a toxic gas with no known useful medical application in specific, adjunctive or preventative therapy. In order for ozone to be effective as a germicide, it must be present in a concentration far greater than that which can be safely tolerated by man.'

The BDA would like more research to take place and to gain assurances that ozone is not harming the mouth. The Association did, however, stress that the use of ozone was a minor issue and that the majority of a dentist's work was now preventive or cosmetic.

NHS reforms

This is definitely the biggest issue in dentistry at present. The UK has two types of dentist that the public can visit, an NHS dentist and a private dentist. Indeed, often the same dentists and dental practices will engage in both types of work. All British citizens are entitled to dental treatment provided by the NHS. This treatment, however, is not free of charge like that received at a GP's surgery. In April 2006, the government introduced new systems of payment for dental treatment, and also changed the way that patients have access to NHS dentists. Under the old system, dentists were paid for each treatment they performed, and there were around 400 separate charges. The new system gives dentists a guaranteed income for providing a certain level of NHS treatment, in order to try to avoid the problem of unnecessary treatment. The payment to dentists is calculated by looking at their income in the period before the reforms came into effect. The government argues that this will take pressure off dentists to treat patients and therefore allow them to spend more time on preventive dentistry.

If you pay for NHS dental treatment, there are three standard charges. Note that you only pay one dental charge even if you need to visit more than once to complete a course of dental treatment. If you need more treatment at the same charge level (e.g. an additional filling) within two months of seeing your dentist, this is free of charge.

NHS dentist charges structure (source: www.whatprice.co.uk/dentist/ nhs-prices.html).

- £16.20 – this charge includes an examination, diagnosis and preventive care. If necessary, this includes X-rays, scale and polish, and planning for further treatment. Urgent and out-of-hours care also costs £16.20.
- £44.60 – this charge includes all necessary treatment covered by the £16.20 charge *plus* additional treatment such as fillings, root canal treatment or extractions.
- £198 – this charge includes all necessary treatment covered by the £16.20 and £44.60 charges *plus* more complex procedures such as crowns, dentures or bridges.
- Repairs to dentures remain free of charge. If you lose or accidentally damage your dentures beyond repair it will cost £56.70 to replace them.
- These charges are valid for any NHS dental treatments finished after 1 April 2008.
- For the period of 1 April 2007 to 1 April 2008 the bands were £15.90, £43.60 and £194, respectively.

Table 5 in Chapter 9 shows a list of different costs, taken from the NHS. You will see in the table that all the procedures listed fit into one of the three bands. A person only pays once – one charge for each course of treatment. For example for a check-up, X-ray, teeth polish, a simple filling and a crown a patient would pay a total of £198 if they all occurred within a two-month period. The drive behind this is for the public to become more conscious of 'preventive dentistry' and to realise that prevention is better than the cure, both in terms of how hard it hits your wallet and how much it hurts once in the dentist's chair. The public is told that ideally people should visit their dentist every six months for a check-up.

The BDA is not particularly happy with the reforms and, as stated in Chapter 6, this is of concern to many dentists. A survey of dentists carried out by the BDA revealed that 55% of dentists did not think that the reforms allowed them to see more patients. Before the reforms, according to the BDA, 32% of dentists performed 95% of their work on NHS patients, but this has fallen to 25% since the reforms. Several dentists have already left, complaining the changes will not end the so-called 'drill and fill' culture. The BDA said the reforms do not give dentists enough time to do preventive work. This has caused strong feelings among dentists, so much so that in some areas up to three-quarters of dentists are threatening to quit the NHS. According to the BDA, the deal states that dentists must carry out 95% of the courses of treatment they currently do to get the same money, which dentists say leaves little time for addressing the causes of poor oral health. Full details of the reforms can be found on the BDA website (www.bda.org).

One dentist I interviewed commented that the NHS does not allow dentists to practise with full clinical freedom and/or reward them for their work, and that until this is sorted out the NHS will remain unattractive to many dentists. As a result many focus on private practice, because private dentistry allows greater clinical freedom and more time with patients. In addition, they are able to use the best materials and laboratories because any earnings can be reinvested into the business/practice and so in the end, both patients and dentists are happier.

It must be remembered that, unlike a doctor, a dentist who runs his or her own practice has costs to meet such as overheads for the premises, wages of staff, materials, new equipment and maintenance, marketing, etc. The NHS structure does not attempt to cover these aspects.

The point to bear in mind as a prospective dentist is to be as informed as possible, not just on this issue but on all of the above, as this will help you to make a better decision with regard to following the course. It will also help to impress a university selection panel at an interview.

Further information

Tables

Table 1: Dental school admissions policies – 2009 entry

	Standard offer	Interview policy	Re-takes considered?	Re-take offer	Sciences preferred
Belfast	AAA + (a) at (AS)	<10%[1]	Yes[2]	AAA + (a) at AS	Two[6,7,8]
Birmingham	AAB	~30–40%	No	–	Two[6,7,9]
Bristol	AAB	~40%	Yes[3]	AAA	Two[6,8,10]
Cardiff	AAB	~40%	Yes	AAA	Two[6]
Dundee	AAA	<40%	No	–	Two[11,12]
Glasgow	AAB	~55%	Yes[3]	AAA	Two[6,11]
King's	AAB + (b) at AS	~40%	Yes[4]	AAB	Two[5,9]
Leeds	AAB	~40–50%	Yes[4]	AAA	Two[6,11]
Liverpool	AAB + (b) at AS	~40%	Yes[3]	AAA	Two[5,9]
Manchester	AAB	~25%	Yes[4]	AAA	Two[6,9,11]
Newcastle	AAB	~20%	No	–	Two[6,11]
Queen Mary	AAB	~60%	Yes[4]	AAA	Three[6,9]
Sheffield	AAB	~40%	Yes[3]	AAA	Two[6,9]

Note: All institutions prefer candidates to have Biology and Chemistry at A level.

1| Interviews are not normally required as part of the selection procedure.
2| Only if you applied first time, held this offer as your first choice and achieved at least ABB + (a) at first attempt.
3| Only if you applied first time, held this offer as your first choice and achieved at least BBB.
4| Only in extenuating circumstances.
5| Two of Chemistry, Biology, Physics, Mathematics or Statistics (one being Chemistry or Biology) at grades AA.
6| Chemistry is required at grade A.
7| Plus at least one from Biology, Physics and Mathematics.
8| Grade A in AS level Biology is required, if not taken at A2 level.
9| If only one of Biology and Chemistry is taken at A level, the other is required at AS level not less than B grades.
10| Biology is essential if the third A level is a non-science subject. Biology should be taken to at least AS level.
11| Biology is required at grade A.
12| Plus two from Chemistry, Physics and Mathematics.

Table 2 (a): Dental school statistics – 2008

	Applications	Interviews	Offers	Accepted
Belfast	163	<10%	74	52
Birmingham	869	304	175	122
Bristol	978	220	194	97
Cardiff	600	175	160	68
Dundee	320	150	142	73
Glasgow	480	260	196	122
King's	967	270	185	128
Leeds	1202	470	202	90
Liverpool*	746	320	240	94
Manchester	876	230	153	76
Newcastle	649	210	200	75
Queen Mary	747	246	167	61
Sheffield	1000	350	220	100

* No new data available at time of writing; entry data for 2006 is given.

Table 2(b): Dental school statistics – 2008

	Clearing	Graduates	Overseas	Re-sits
Belfast	0	4	0	9
Birmingham	0	6	2	0
Bristol	0	11	2	2
Cardiff	4	1	4	6
Dundee	0	3	3	0
Glasgow	0	0	3	0
King's	0	15	10	0
Leeds	0	7	8	6
Liverpool*	0	16	4	0
Manchester	0	6	4	4
Newcastle	0	7	6	0
Queen Mary	0	4	5	5
Sheffield	0	2	4	6

* No new data available at time of writing; entry data for 2006 is given.

Table 3: Typical interviews

	Length	Number on panel	Composition of panel	Written element?
Belfast	20 min	Three	Director of the Centre for Dental Education, plus an academic staff member, and academic related staff member	No
Birmingham	15 min	Two	Admissions tutor plus an academic staff member	No
Bristol	20 min	Two	Clinical and non-clinical staff	Essay response to a dental-related topic
Cardiff	15 min	Two	At least one senior clinician	No
Dundee	20 min	Two	Academic and clinical staff	No
Glasgow	20 min	Three	Two members of admission committee (qualified dentists) and an administrator	Yes – portfolio document is sent out and the applicant has to respond to its various demands
King's	20 min	Two	Admissions tutor plus another academic	Questionnaire and ethical case study
Leeds	15 min	Three	One academic, one clinical academic and one student	No
Liverpool	15 min	Two	Members of academic staff and local GDPs	No
Manchester	15 min	Two/ three	Members of clinical and non-clinical teaching staff	No
Newcastle	20 min	Two	Senior members of academic staff (at least one clinician)	No
Queen Mary	30 min	Three	One academic, one clinician and one student	Yes – DVD shown and responses elicited from student
Sheffield	15 min	Two	One clinician member of staff and a second from another department or a community dentist	No

Table 4: Applicants through UCAS to dentistry by the October deadline

Applicants		UK			Other EU		
		Men	Women	Total	Men	Women	Total
Dentistry	2009	1,287	1,558	2,845	70	120	190
	2008	1,209	1,388	2,597	70	112	182
	% change	6.45%	12.25%	9.55%	0.00%	7.14%	4.40%
	Difference	78	170	248	0	8	8

	Non-EU			All		
	Men	Women	Total	Men	Women	Total
2009	93	176	269	1,450	1,854	3,304
2008	80	136	216	1,359	1,636	2,995
% change	16.25%	29.41%	24.54%	6.70%	13.33%	10.32%
Difference	13	40	53	91	218	309

Source: www.ucas.ac.uk/website/news/media_releases/2008/2008-10-28

Table 5: Dental procedure costs

Dental work required	NHS prices
Apicoectomy	£198.00
Braces	£198.00
Dental crown	£198.00
Dental examination	£16.20
Dentures	£198.00
First consultation	£16.20
Large tooth filling	£121.30
Root canal	£198.00
Sedated tooth removal	£44.60
Small tooth filling	£44.60
Scale and polish	£16.20
X-ray	£16.20

Source: www.whatprice.co.uk/dentist/nhs-prices.html
Note: NHS dentist treatment is completely free if you are:

- under 18
- 18 but in full-time education
- pregnant or have given birth within the last 12 months
- receiving income support, job-seeker's allowance or 'guarantee credit' on your pension credit – or your partner is receiving one of these.

Postgraduate deaneries in the UK

South and East

Anglia
Postgraduate Medical and Dental Education
East Anglia Deanery
Block 3, Ida Darwin Site
Fulbourn Hospital
Cambridge
CB1 5EE
Tel: 01223 884847

Thames
Department of Postgraduate Dentistry
Thames Postgraduate Medical and Dental Education
33 Millman Street
London
WC1N 3EJ
Tel: 020 7692 3148

Oxford
Oxford Postgraduate Medical and Dental Education
The Triangle
Roosevelt Drive
Headington
Oxford
OX3 7XP
Tel: 01865 740650

Wessex
Postgraduate Dean's Department
NHS Executive South and West (Wessex Deanery)
Highcroft
Romsey Road
Winchester
SO22 5DH
Tel: 01962 863511, extension 205

North

Scotland
Scottish Council for Postgraduate Medical and Dental Education
4th Floor, Hobart House
80 Hanover Street
Edinburgh
EH2 1EL
Tel: 0131 225 4365

Northern Ireland
Northern Ireland Council for Postgraduate Medical and Dental Education
5 Annadale Avenue
Belfast
BT7 3JH
Tel: 028 9049 4809

Mersey
Department of Postgraduate Dental Education and Training
Ground Floor
Hamilton House
24 Pall Mall
Liverpool
L3 6AL
Tel: 0151 285 2265

Northern
Postgraduate Institute for Medicine and Dentistry
10–12 Framlington Place
Newcastle upon Tyne
NE2 4AB
Tel: 0191 222 7908

North Western
The North Western Deanery
4th Floor, Barlow House
Minshull Street
Manchester
M1 3DZ
Tel: 0161 237 3690

Yorkshire
The Department for NHS Postgraduate Medical and Dental Education
Willow Terrace Road
University of Leeds
Leeds LS2 9JT
Tel: 0113 233 1526

West

South West
Dental Postgraduate Department
Bristol Dental Hospital
Lower Maudlin Street
Bristol
BS1 2LY
Tel: 0117 928 4522

Trent
Regional Postgraduate Dental Office
The University of Sheffield
Medical School
Beech Hill Road
Sheffield
S10 2RX
Tel: 0114 271 7983

Wales
Postgraduate Office
Room 155
Dental School
Heath Park
Cardiff
CF4 4XY
Tel: 029 2074 3649 / 2594

West Midlands
Postgraduate Office
The Dental School
St Chad's Queensway
Birmingham
B4 6NN
Tel: 0121 237 2830/2831

Source: UCL Eastman Dental Institute (www.eastman.ucl.ac.uk/education/careerguide/index.html)

■ Further reading

An essential starting point is the BDA's website (www.bda.org). This carries careers information for prospective dentists as well as press releases and discussion of topical issues. The BDA's websites for dental patients (www.bdasmile.org and http://bda-findadentist.org.uk) are also useful.

The BDA has its own museum, the BDA Dental Museum. Details can be found at www.bda.org/museum. An entertaining (and informative) site is www.3dmouth.org which contains, as the name suggests, a computer-generated three-dimensional mouth.

The BDA publishes a journal for dentists, the *British Dental Journal*. Again, details of this appear on the BDA website. The journal is aimed at practising dentists, and can be very technical. More accessible is *Launchpad*, the BDA's magazine for dental students and newly qualified dentists.

Dentistry (www.dentistry.co.uk) is an independent dental magazine published every fortnight. It carries news, clinical articles, business articles, education features and product information.

To keep up to date with dentistry and dental issues in the UK, the *Independent*, the *Guardian*, the *Daily Telegraph* and *The Times* all carry regular health reporting, and have health sections once a week. The Sunday broadsheet papers often contain summaries of medicine- or dentistry-related issues.

Another source of dental news is the website www.topix.net/business/dental, which covers topical dentistry stories from the UK and worldwide.

For information on grade requirements, see *Degree Course Offers*, written by Brian Heap and published by Trotman (www.trotman.co.uk; tel: 020 8486 1150), or the *UCAS Big Guide* (UCAS, tel: 01242 222444).

If you are thinking of studying dentistry overseas, M&D Europe is a good source of information. It aims to help you get a place on a course taught in English – and, once you have qualified, to help you get placements at hospitals in the UK. Its website, www.readmedicine.com, gives details of dental schools in the Czech Republic and the Cayman Islands.

The International Society for Fluoride Research publishes its own journal called *Fluoride*. Some articles from the journal are available on the society's website (www.fluoride-journal.com). Queen Mary's *Rough Guide to Dentistry* can be accessed on its website (www.qmul.ac.uk/medicineanddentistry). www.admissionsforum.net is a chatroom for potential medical and dental applicants.

Contact details

Organisations

British Dental Association
64 Wimpole Street
London
W1G 8YS
Tel: 0207 935 0875
Website: www.bda.org

British Fluoridation Society
4th Floor, School of Dentistry
University of Liverpool
Liverpool
L69 3BX
Email: bfs@liv.ac.uk

British Medical Association
BMA House
Tavistock Square
London
WC1H 9JP
Tel: 020 7387 4499
Website: www.bma.org.uk

General Dental Council
37 Wimpole Street
London
W1G 8DQ
Tel: 020 7887 3800
Website: www.gdc-uk.org

Dental schools

BELFAST
Mrs Dwyer, Admissions Tutor

Queen's University
Grosvenor Road
Belfast
BT12 6BP
Tel: 028 9097 2727
Fax: 028 9042 8861
Website: www.qub.ac.uk

BIRMINGHAM
Mr Donald Spence, Admissions Tutor
Ms Keeley Turner, Admission Secretary

School of Dentistry
University of Birmingham
St Chad's Queensway
Birmingham
B4 6NN
Tel: 0121 237 2761
Fax: 0121 625 8815
Website: www.dentistry.bham.ac.uk

BRISTOL
Dr John Moran, Admissions Tutor
Ms Geraldine Vines, Admissions Secretary

Dental School
University of Bristol
Lower Maudlin Street

Bristol
BS1 2LY
Tel: 0117 928 4307
Fax: 0117 928 4150
Website: www.dentalschool.bris.ac.uk

CARDIFF
Mrs Victoria J Ocock, Admissions Officer

Dental School
Cardiff University
Heath Park
Cardiff
CF14 4XY
Tel: 029 2074 6917
Fax: 029 2076 6343
Website: www.cardiff.ac.uk/dentistry

DUNDEE
Mr Gordon Black, Admissions Tutor
Mrs Carol Boag, Information Assistant

Admissions & Student Recruitment
University of Dundee
Nethergate
Dundee
DD1 4HN
Tel (direct): 01382 383838
Fax: 01382 385500
Email: c.z.boag@dundee.ac.uk
Website: www.dundee.ac.uk/admissions

GLASGOW
Dr Christine Goodall, Admissions Tutor
Mr Stewart Hutchinson, Deputy Admissions Officer

Glasgow Dental Hospital and School
378 Sauchiehall Street
Glasgow
G2 3JZ
Tel: 0141 211 9703/4
Fax: 0141 331 2798
Website: www.gla.ac.uk/schools/dental

KING'S COLLEGE LONDON
Dr Cabot, Admissions Officer

Guy's, King's & St Thomas' Dental Institute
King's College London
Hodgkin Building
Guy's Campus

London
SE1 1UL
Tel: 020 7848 6512
Fax: 020 7848 6510
Website: www.kcl.ac.uk/depsta/dentistry

LEEDS
Dr Simon Wood, Admissions Tutor
Miss Helen Russell, Undergraduate Administrator

Leeds Dental Institute
Leeds University
Clarendon Way
Leeds
LS2 9LU
Tel: 0113 343 6199
Email: h.c.russell@leeds.ac.uk
Website: www.leeds.ac.uk/dental

LIVERPOOL
Miss Eileen Theil, Admissions Tutor
Miss Abbey Watkins, Admissions Secretary

School of Dentistry
University of Liverpool
Pembroke Place
Liverpool
L3 5PS
Tel: 0151 706 5298
Fax: 0151 706 5652
Website: www.liv.ac.uk/dental

MANCHESTER
Dr Tony Mellor, Admissions Tutor
Mrs Teresa Smith, Undergraduate Admissions Secretary (BDS)

Dean's Administrative Offices
University Dental Hospital of Manchester
Higher Cambridge Street
Manchester
M15 6FH
Tel: 0161 306 0231
Fax: 0161 306 0221
Website: www.den.man.ac.uk

NEWCASTLE
Mrs L O'Connor, School Administrator

School of Dental Sciences
Framlington Place
Newcastle University

Newcastle upon Tyne
NE2 4BW
Tel: 0191 222 8347
Fax: 0191 222 6137
Website: www.ncl.ac.uk/dental

PENINSULA COLLEGE OF MEDICINE AND DENTISTRY
Sue Cook, Senior Admissions Coordinator

Peninsula Dental School
John Bull Building
Tamar Science Park
Plymouth
PL6 8BU
Tel: 01752 437333
Fax: 01752 517842
Website: www.pms.ac.uk

QUEEN MARY (BARTS AND THE LONDON)
Dr Chris Mercer, Admissions Tutor
Ms Natasha Chapel, Admissions Secretary

St Bartholomew's and the Royal London School of Medicine and
Dentistry
Garrod Building
Turner Street
London
E1 2AD
Tel: 0207 882 2243
Fax: 0207 882 7284
Website: www.smd.qmul.ac.uk/dental

SHEFFIELD
Mrs Amanda Okrasa, Admissions Secretary

The School of Clinical Dentistry
The University of Sheffield
Claremont Crescent
Sheffield
S10 2TA
Tel: 0114 271 7808
Fax: 0114 279 7050
Website: www.shef.ac.uk/dentalschool